Gastric Sleeve Bariatric Surgery Cookbook

The Complete Guide to Achieving Weight Loss Surgery Success with Over 100 Delicious Healthy Recipes

Kristin Scott

Table of Contents

4

5

The following Book is reproduced below with the goal of providing information that is as accurate and reliable as possible. Regardless, purchasing this Book can be seen as consent to the fact that both the publisher and the author of this book are in no way experts on the topics discussed within and that any recommendations or suggestions that are made herein are for entertainment purposes only. Professionals should be consulted as needed prior to undertaking any of the action endorsed herein.

This declaration is deemed fair and valid by both the American Bar Association and the Committee of Publishers Association and is legally binding throughout the United States.

Furthermore, the transmission, duplication or reproduction of any of the following work including specific information will be considered an illegal act irrespective of if it is done electronically or in print. This extends to creating a secondary or tertiary copy of the work or a recorded copy and is only allowed with an expressed written consent from the Publisher. All additional rights reserved.

The information in the following pages is broadly considered to be truthful and accurate account of facts, and as such any inattention, use or misuse of the information in question by the reader will render any resulting actions solely under their purview. There are no scenarios in which the publisher or the original author of this work can be in any fashion deemed liable for any hardship or damages that may befall them after undertaking information described herein.

Additionally, the information in the following pages is intended only for informational purposes and should thus be thought of as universal. As befitting its nature, it is presented without assurance regarding its prolonged validity or interim quality. Trademarks that are mentioned are done without written consent and can in no way be considered an endorsement from the trademark holder.

Introduction

Congratulations on purchasing *"Gastric Sleeve Bariatric Surgery Cookbook: The Complete Guide to Achieving Weight Loss Surgery Success with Over 100 Delicious Healthy Recipes"* and thank you for doing so. It is my pleasure to help you on this journey.

The following chapters will offer you a supportive overview of what exactly a Vertical Sleeve Gastrectomy is and what you can expect before, during, and after this procedure. If this is a journey you have chosen to take with the goal towards a healthier quality of living, then this is the book written to assist you as you work towards your goals.

The information in this book is derived from no medical source earlier than 2017 and covers a wide base of scientific research and medical consensus. The road to renewed health is a never-ending journey of discovery in which the opportunities available to you, post-surgery, are infinite. The decision you have made to undergo a Sleeve Gastrectomy is not a frivolous decision. You have committed to changing your life. This book is written with your decision in mind. All of the information contained within these pages will help assist you in making the correct choices moving forward.

Along with the science-based evidence that a Gastric Sleeve surgery will improve your health, we have also noted the practical steps you will need to take along the way. A review of a possible pre-procedure diet, a 4-week post-surgery diet insight, 2-week post-surgery meal plan, plenty of delicious recipes, exercises, non-surgical options for firming and tightening your skin once you have lost the weight, a plan on how and when to buy your new wardrobe, and plenty more!

Every effort was made to ensure this book is full of useful

information for you. Your success is important to everyone. Let's get started.

Chapter 1: Gastric Sleeve Surgery Basics

Vertical Sleeve Gastrectomy

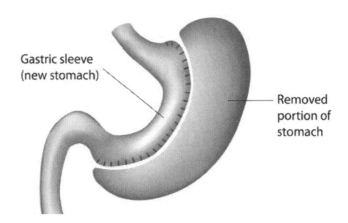

Vertical Sleeve Gastrectomy

Vertical Sleeve Gastrectomy or also known as Gastric Sleeve surgery is not for the faint of heart. I commend you for taking the active step to a healthier life. This choice should not be taken lightly as it involves a radical re-adjustment of many patterns of behavior, both conscious and unconscious. Preparing yourself with as much information as possible before surgery will vastly increase your ability to create a successful transition into a new healthier lifestyle. It is important for you to realize; the surgery must be considered as a 'tool' in your weight loss journey and not a 'quick fix.' Your success with this journey will also depend on other important factors such as mindset, mental discipline, exercise, nutritional education, change of habits, and modifying your behavior among other things.

History

Originally, this procedure was used to modify another weight loss surgery, the duodenal switch. It continued to develop over time and was later used as phase one in a two-phase bypass operation on patients suffering from extreme obesity, which could not undertake the risk of the regular procedure. The patients experiencing the phase one operation were so successful with their initial loss of weight that doctors began to investigate the potential of phase one as a procedure all on its own.

What is it?

The Gastric Sleeve procedure is a permanent non-reversible surgery, resulting in a much smaller stomach. For many individuals, the surgeon will choose to perform the procedure laparoscopically, incising several neat openings in your abdomen of approximately 1/4 to 1/2 inches in length. A laparoscope is then inserted, a uniquely sized tool complete with light and camera which is hooked up to a nearby computer. Photographs of the surgery are then displayed in real time on the monitor for your surgeon to make informed choices on how best to proceed during the operation.

The surgeon will then reduce the stomach to approximately 20 percent of its original size (depending on the patient) by surgically removing a large section along its curvature as you can see in the image above. The resulting shape is a tubular or sleeve-like apparatus. This new stomach will continue to fill the same distance from esophagus to intestine. The original outlet or pyloric valve will continue to operate in its normal function, releasing food from the newly created sleeve to the small intestine.

Consequently, this reduces the amount of food needed to feel full, significantly. Not only does this procedure increase the feeling of satiation with much smaller amounts of food, but it also decreases the feeling of hunger. How? You may ask. Well, the large part of the stomach that is removed contains the highest concentration of the cells that release the hunger hormone, known as "ghrelin." So, throughout the day, you will notice that your desire for food will be a lot less. Furthermore, daily calorie consumption will naturally decrease substantially, resulting in serious weight loss over time.

How does this method differ from a bypass surgery procedure?

The method, known as a stomach or bariatric bypass operation, is the most commonly used procedure in the United States for surgery as a means of weight loss. Like the Gastric Sleeve procedure, in many instances, bypass surgery is irreversible. The surgery itself with a bypass requires a slight increase in the amount of time to perform. The Gastric Sleeve takes approximately an hour while the Bypass requires about 1.5 hours. Both surgeries require two to three days in hospital post-surgery (barring no complications arise), and a 2-4 week recovery period.

With the Bypass procedure, a surgeon may opt to use laparoscopy, similar to the Gastric Sleeve procedure, or they may make one 10-12 inch incision in the abdomen. The stomach itself is assessed, and a pouch is built along the top. The pouch area is defined by the insertion of surgical staples. This pocket will eventually be capable of holding up to one cup of food. An average stomach can hold up to 6 cups of food.

The surgeon then must attach the small intestine to this 'new' stomach which requires the food to move directly to the mid-section of their small intestine, bypassing the rest of the stomach and its connection to the upper area of the small intestine. They then must join the upper small intestine to its mid-section, allowing for the flow of digestive fluids from the lower stomach to flow down from the upper

13

small intestine into the mid-section of the intestine. The incision will then be closed by staples or stitches.

What are the qualifications for the surgery?

As there are inherent risks when it comes to any type of surgery, you will likely need to go through an extensive screening process before being cleared for a Sleeve Gastrectomy. Generally speaking, you may qualify to move forward in this way if you:

- Find your efforts to lose weight via traditional means are unsuccessful
- Your body mass index is 40 or above
- Your body mass index is at a minimum of 35, and you have one or more serious weight-related health issues such as severe sleep apnea, high blood pressure or type 2 diabetes
- Some people with extremely severe enough weight-based health issues may also qualify for the surgery even if their body mass index is between 30 and 34.
- Are a teenager who has been through puberty, an adult between the ages of 18 and 60, or you are over the age of 60 and in otherwise good health.

In addition to the guidelines outlined above, you should also expect to be analyzed by a medical team that includes a surgeon, dietitian, doctor, and a psychologist who will determine if you are a good candidate for surgery. This evaluation will weigh the benefits you will see from the surgery as well as both the mental and physical challenges you may face along the way. One unexpected disqualifying factor for many people is depressive or suicidal thoughts as there is an increased risk of suicide among those who have had the procedure, though the reasons as to why this is the case are not yet clear.

While having a history of depressive or suicidal thoughts do not, necessarily, mean you cannot have the surgery, it will mean that your health care team will need to carefully evaluate your plan for the future as well as your medical history before clearing you for surgery. Additionally, they will look more closely at your weight and nutrition history including things like motivation for the surgery, time constraints, average stress level, exercise and eating habits, common weight trends and previous diet attempts.

As issues like nutritional deficiencies, kidney stones, heart problems, liver disease, and blood clots can all increase the inherent risks of surgery, your health care team will also evaluate your current medical condition if you drink or smoke, the types of medications you take. There are also several mental conditions that can harm your application process or even lead to disqualification including; issues arising from sexual abuse, severe bipolar disorder, schizophrenia, major depression, anxiety disorders, substance abuse, and binge-eating disorder.

What are the benefits of a Sleeve Gastrectomy?

- This type of surgery is ideal for those who have a difficult time controlling themselves around food as it takes willpower of the equation completely. As it leaves your pylorus in place, it also allows you to feel full normally, despite consuming far fewer calories than what was likely once the case.

- Through the reduction in the size of your stomach, you will be restricted to eating smaller amounts of food, which in turn creates a feeling of fullness or satiation much sooner. By consuming fewer calories, you will lose weight. Up to 60 or 70 percent of your excess weight will be lost in a 12-18 month post-operation period.

- Your desire to eat will be less because the surgery removes the part of your stomach that is mostly responsible for producing ghrelin, which is responsible for making you feel hungry.

- The weight loss will improve or can even cure some of the related conditions you have been suffering as a result of being obese. These conditions include high blood pressure, diabetes (Type 2), and diseases of the cardiopulmonary system. Reducing your weight can often decrease the number of medications required to treat any weight-related conditions.

- Other positive health outcomes attributed to Gastric Sleeve surgery include a longer lifespan. A large study of the population compared bariatric and non-bariatric surgical patients and discovered an over 90 percent reduced death rate from diabetes and more than 50 percent reduced rate of dying from heart-related diseases.

- Patients can also enjoy relief and even cessation of the following diseases related to obesity: breathing associated disorders, urinary incontinence, reflux disease, disorders caused by high blood pressure, sleep apnea, abnormal cholesterol, liver disease, dangers of blood clots and many more. Depression and anxiety are two mental illnesses which are notably reduced following surgery.

- Finally, a Sleeve Gastrectomy can cause a substantial improvement in your quality of life. The medical profession measures quality of life through evaluating your social interactions, personal self-esteem, ability to work, and through the development of personal relationships. Higher energy levels lead to increased participation in activities which bring you into direct communication with others, for example, swimming, walking, and bike riding. Friendships are developed, leading to positive feedback for the activity and creating an increased desire to continue the activity. Positive social interactions boost a person's self-esteem, leading to a potential increase in personal relationships.

- Unlike with more traditional bypass surgery, the bowel is not subject to any rearrangement which means that dumping, which is often known to occur in bypass patients when the contents of their stomachs are dumped into their small intestines too quickly, is very unlikely to occur.

What are the risks associated with the procedure?

- Vomiting if you accidentally eat more than your new stomach can hold
- Scar tissue can form on the inside of your stomach, which could eventually lead to a blockage of the bowel if left untreated.
- Increased risk of stomach ulcers, heartburn, or inflammation of the stomach lining.
- Leakage of digestive juices along the staple line of the stomach which can lead to serious infections.

How to find success after the surgery?

While having the surgery will certainly give you a leg up when it comes to finding weight loss success moving forward, the fact of the matter is that it is only the first step in what needs to be a dramatic lifestyle change. The truth is approximately 30 percent of patients after bariatric surgery start to gain their weight back after the initial honeymoon post-surgery time period. This weight gain is due to the sleeve having the stomach tissue's resilient feature of being able to stretch. Without attention to good choices being made in your diet, the stomach can and will stretch back to its pre-surgery size. If you want to find true success after the surgery, here are a few tips.

- One way to prepare you for post-operative success is to start initiating good lifestyle patterns before the surgery. These pattern changing ideas include locating a surgical weight loss support group close by your home and joining up before surgery. This will provide you with a network of friends who can offer pre- and post-op advice and share some coping strategies with you. Challenges and achievements can be shared with others who have personal experience with the surgery process. There are also some programs which invite family members to become involved, creating a patient's in-house support program.

- You can sign up for a nutritional counseling class or one-on-one private sessions. Learn up-to-date factual information about food and adequate nutrition. Do not listen to unverified claims when it comes to your personal dietary needs.

- Try to stop any binge-eating patterns you may have long before you have the surgery. Visit a therapist or counselor to discuss why these patterns might exist and what you need to do to enact change. Binge-eating occurrences are related to issues we may be carrying with us from our childhood. If you want to change your behaviors, you will need to address why they exist in the first place. This can also be said for any alcohol or drug dependencies you might have. All three of these are symptoms of a problem and not the problem itself.

- Follow your doctor's advice to the letter both before and after the surgery. They are the professional, and there are well-documented reasons for why they are requesting you to do certain things. Don't be afraid to ask questions; information will enable you to make the right choices confidently.

- Finally, if after the surgery you feel unwell, address this with your doctor right away. To feel good about the changes you are going through, you need to know that what you are experiencing is normal and as it should be. This is a brand new body you are creating and the more information you have available to you, the more confident you will be that each step you take on your journey is the right one for you.

- There is one more area that is very important to address post-surgery – your emotional well-being. Electing to have a Sleeve Gastrectomy is a very important decision in your life. The resulting physical and energetic changes will affect other's perceptions of you as well as your perceptions of yourself. You need to know that this choice you made is for your health and quality of life.

- Counseling is often recommended for patients both before and after the surgery to protect their emotional health. Having an opportunity to receive counseling, both pre- and post-surgery allows them to build realistic expectations around what to expect both from themselves and their loved ones. It is very important for everyone involved to navigate the changes which occur as a result of a bariatric procedure.

- Creating a strong and positive mindset. As your body starts to change, you will also need to make an effort to develop a strong and positive mindset. This is super important, as your mindset will be what keeps you on track to achieving your goals and preventing a relapse.

While the patient may experience a life-altering positive effect after surgery, the changes will ripple down through family and friends, affecting everyone involved differently. Many obese people prefer to be out of the social radar, and after years of avoiding notice, you will now become a spotlighted figure for the dramatic change you incur. This can be tough to adjust too, and having someone who can offer professional advice will be required.

Ultimately you have made this choice for you. In doing this, you have said, 'Hey, I am an individual of value. I matter enough to make sure I live a long, healthy life.' A Gastric Sleeve Bariatric procedure can be life-changing. And like all changes that enhance our lives, we need to respect the changes taking place and allow them time and attention to achieve fruition.

Chapter 2: The 4 Phases of the Gastric Sleeve Diet

In preparation for your surgery, your doctor will provide you with a specific diet to follow. This diet is tailored to your specific needs and nutritional requirements. As your doctor knows what's best, follow what they prescribe.

What I can tell you about the primary goal for this pre-surgery meal regime is to shrink your liver. Your liver has probably accumulated an excess of fat cells both around and inside of it. The liver is located right next to your stomach, and an overly large liver can make the Sleeve Gastrectomy procedure much harder to achieve.

In preparation, the doctor will usually assign you a diet plan two weeks before your surgery date. This diet is very strict, intending to reduce your overall caloric intake through a reduction in carbohydrates (pasta, sweets, potatoes). You will follow a diet that consists of foods you will be eating post-surgery. You can think of this time period as a good introduction to the foods you will be developing an intimate relationship with post-surgery. These food friends include lean proteins, vegetables, and no to low-calorie drinks. You may even be assigned a daily calorie goal for this time period.

You can check to see if any of the recipes in Chapter 5 match with the meals on your diet plan and find out which ones you really like and maybe ones you do not wish to maintain a relationship with.

The two days before your operation, you will be asked to consume a diet of clear liquids only. This might include a single sugarless protein beverage a day along with clear broth, decaffeinated tea or coffee, popsicles without sugar and everyone's favorite hospital food, gelatin. No caffeinated beverages will be allowed.

This is a basic outline of what you can expect diet-wise before your Sleeve Gastrectomy procedure. I have listed the breakdown of what to expect and achieve in your diet over days and weeks after your surgery. The transitioning changes in the body's physical requirements to achieve the best outcome post-op have been mapped out over four distinct phases. You might transition from one phase to the next a little earlier or a little later than what is defined here. Be patient and alert to what your body needs. The phases are designed to assist in your transition to a healthier version of you which you can enjoy for the rest of your life.

It is vital that should you have any concerns or questions that you do not hesitate to contact your doctor for assistance.

Phase 1: Day 1 - 7

Immediately following the operation, most patients feel very little or no hunger for the first few days. It is VERY IMPORTANT to remain well-hydrated. This can speed up the process of healing and ease any feelings of nausea or vomiting.

Clear liquids only are allowed. At least eight glasses of water per day should be consumed. The following are also acceptable; broth, sugarless jello, decaffeinated coffee or tea, and sugarless popsicles.

It is important to be aware that absolutely no consumption of beverages with caffeine in them are allowed, along with drinks with sugar like fruit juices, soda pops, or carbonated beverages.

Phase 2: Day 7 - 14

You might start to notice an increase in your appetite during this time period. This is natural and only to be expected. However, do not take this as a reason for consuming solid foods. Your digestive tract is not able to handle this kind of responsibility yet. Eating solid foods could lead to complications such as vomiting or worse. Maintaining the no sugar and fat rule while drinking liquids will assist with your preparedness for the next stage of the diet. Continue to avoid caffeine and carbonated drinks.

You now require a fuller liquid diet, that is protein rich. Your goal here is to consume a wide variety of healthy nutrients while avoiding foods containing little to no nutritional density. Continue to drink water, a lot of it, as well as milk, broth, and sugar-free juice.

You should start to include some protein powder in your diet.

23

The powder should be free of sugar and only mix it with full or clear liquid. You should aim to consume 20g of protein daily while limiting yourself to 250ml of liquid each meal.

Foods you can now incorporate into your diet include thin soups, sugar-free pudding, juice that has been diluted, sugar-free instant breakfasts, soft noodles, fat and sugar-free ice cream or yogurt or sorbet, applesauce with no sugar can be diluted with water before eating.

Foods that should still be avoided include all foods with sugar, foods with high-fat content, and chunky foods.

Phase 3: Day 14 – 28

It is at this phase where it is safe to start incorporating thicker pureed foods. Take the time to ensure they are well-cooked and soft before consuming. Anything low in fat and free of sugar which you can puree can be eaten at this point. It will become very important to start increasing your protein intake as well. If the taste of pureed meat makes you uncomfortable, stick to the shakes with no sugar and begin to eat eggs.

You should now be aiming for up to 60-80 grams of protein a day. Foods rich in protein appropriate for this phase include scrambled eggs, yogurt (Greek), pureed chicken, and fish. It is best to make sure you are ingesting enough protein, so try to consume that first in each meal. Other foods that are now safe to consume include; low or no sugar baby foods, thinned oatmeal, low or no sugar smoothies, mashed potatoes, and sweet potatoes. It is important to note that each meal should not exceed more than half a cup. As a result, many small meals will be required.

After a few days to a week in phase 3, you can now start to transition from pureed-like foods to soft foods. You must continue consuming approximately 60g – 80g of protein daily. Nutrient dense foods you can now start to add to your diet, in addition to the foods from the previous phases include; boiled eggs, soft fish, low-fat cheese and deli meat, very soft vegetables (no skin), thicker soups (can have some chunks). You may want to continue drinking a low sugar protein shake to ensure you are meeting your required daily protein intake.

Chunky, solid foods should continue to be avoided along with spices. The latter may lead to heartburn. Bland food with little or no seasoning is best. Foods you must still stay away from include; anything with high sugar, anything high in fat, bread, tough vegetables, white pasta, white rice.

You may be allowed to incorporate 1-2 cups of coffee if your Doctor approves.

Phase 4 – Transitioning to Solid Foods: Day 28 and onwards

You are now roughly one-month post-procedure and ready for the introduction of solid foods back into your diet providing your Doctor confirms this. Here is where your healthy eating habits start to begin. You will continue to require 60 - 80g of protein each day and will most likely need to consume a low sugar protein shake to help reach this target. Continue your path of good hydration but remember to stop drinking 30 minutes before meals and not to drink anything until 30 minutes afterward. You also want to stick to the daily regime of 3 meals, two snacks.

Caffeinated drinks should be fine at this time but continue to stay away from carbonated beverages such as soda pop. Remember, you do not have many calories to work with. You want to ensure you are spending your very limited amount of calories on foods that are very high in nutrients and make you feel satiated. If you spend your very limited amount of calories on foods and drinks that are not nutritious, it will lead to nutritional deficiencies. Now that your stomach size is much smaller, you have to be much wiser on what foods you consume.

Foods you can now bring into the diet include; low fat cottage cheese, small amounts of fruit, fish, lean meats, and vegetables.

Continue to avoid high fat and sugar-dense foods. This includes anything packaged or fried. These foods are high in calories and offer

26

no nutritional value to you. You also want to continue to avoid white grains and bread.

Exercise

This depends on the individual, and when your Doctor thinks it is safe for you to start exercising. Regular exercise will be a great addition to your new healthy lifestyle and will accelerate your weight loss progress. Your Doctor may start you off on light, less strenuous exercising such as walking and yoga before progressing you to higher strenuous activities like weight lifting.

Mindset

Mindset is not something to underestimate. Mindset is equally as important as diet and exercise. Along your journey to a new healthier version of you, make an effort to improve your state of mind and perception of things. Your mindset will play a big role in your weight loss success, and it's something you can start improving today! Mindset will be one of the few things that carry you through the hard times of diet and exercise.

When you may experience difficulty on a diet, your mindset will be the helping hand when you are faced with moments of temptation. Your mindset will help you fight against temptation and continue to stay on track towards the desired end goal. Each time you do this and resist temptation, your will-power will ultimately become stronger too. When you are faced with difficulty during your workouts, and things are getting tough, and you feel like you want to give up, your mindset will be the one thing that helps you push through those moments of pain and progress towards the desired end goal.

Do not underestimate the power of a strong mind. Make conscious efforts to improve your mindset and perspective. Start listening to positive and encouraging things. Surround yourself with positive and uplifting people who have strong mindsets. This will ultimately help you greatly towards your transformation.

Chapter 3: Nutritional Concerns

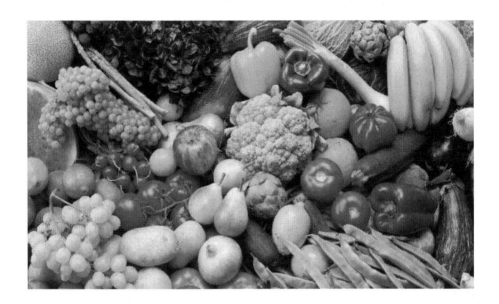

Guidelines for eating following surgery

A big part of maintaining the healthy lifestyle changes you will see after your surgery in the long-term is ensuring that when you do eat, you eat the right things. This chapter will discuss the types of foods you should prioritize, as well as provide a meal plan based on the recipes found in Chapter 5. This material does not replace what a trained health professional can offer but provides a general overview of what is generally prescribed and perhaps give you a little more insight into what the professionals are talking about.

Before we get into definitions and listings of nutrient-rich foods, let's review the guidelines for eating following surgery.

- Consume three light meals a day as well as 1-2 snacks if you feel the need. This should include breakfast. This will total to eating a maximum of 5 times during the day.

- Take the time to eat your food slowly. You have a new smaller stomach, so you need to be careful.

- You need to limit your food consumption to 250 ml or 1 cup (approximately) of food for each meal.

- Choose mostly solid foods with high nutritional value during these meals.

- Foods that are tricky to chew, for example, foods that are tough, stringy, doughy, or very sticky, should be avoided as these can create discomfort and even vomiting. This is due to the obstruction in the pouch stoma (stomach opening).

- Fluids should only be consumed more than thirty minutes before and thirty minutes after eating solid foods.

- All liquids and liquid foods (i.e., soups) can be enjoyed between the consumption of solid food.

- Soda pops or any carbonated drink should not be consumed. This is a waste of calories that provides no nutritional value to your body.

- Do not consume foods or drinks with a high sugar content to assist in the prevention of Dumping Syndrome. This Syndrome is a group of symptoms which can occur in some patients after the surgery when they eat. Discomfort in the abdominal area, weakness, and occasionally very rapid emptying of the bowels.

- Remember to take any prescribed vitamins and supplements. Generally, this will include one multi-vitamin, a mineral supplement, and perhaps some extra calcium and Vitamin D if necessary.

- Consume approximately 60-80g of protein daily. If you are struggling to reach this amount of protein per day, you should have a low sugar protein shake daily to reach the required protein amount.

Remember that you have worked extremely hard to arrive at this place in your life. It is best to consider the above recommendations as a lifelong pattern and not a temporary measure. Patterns of behavior are created through repetition, and in the beginning, you will need to focus on the pattern created to avoid any negative behaviors creeping in.

The following lists are behaviors that can cause gradual weight gain and behaviors you must avoid. They may start as small as one or two-time indulgences that can increase in frequency through the months ahead. Stay vigilant about your goals for a healthy life.

Weight gain happens when:

- You start to choose foods which are dense in calories and not in nutrients.
- You increase how often you eat in a day. Eating more than five times a day is too many.
- You begin to 'nibble' between meals.
- You start to consume foods high in fat
- You start to consume foods high in sugar
- You start consuming drinks with more calories than what should be in your overall calorie goal for the day.
- Drinking soda pop or other high sugar carbonated drinks.
- You begin to ignore the thirty-minute rule about drinking pre and post meals.
- You are constantly over-consuming in one sitting and stretching your stomach.

Avoid these behavioral patterns at all costs. If you can feel yourself slipping into bad habits, you need to improve your mindset and re-align yourself with the desired end goal and why you want to achieve this goal. The notion of 'just this once' must be deferred indefinitely when it comes to eating and drinking.

Now let's look at what to eat.

Nutrient dense foods can be defined as food that is relatively low in calories and high in nutrients. When we consider what a nutrient is, these are foods that contain high amounts of vitamins and minerals. They are rich in complex carbohydrates, contain lean proteins, and only the healthy type of fats.

There are many foods that fit this description. Some foods can amp up your nutrient consumption without increasing your overall caloric intake. These foods, such as fruits and vegetables, are the direct opposite of what is known as 'calorie-dense' foods.

Nutrient density can be used to distinguish different kinds of foods from each other, oatmeal versus frosted flakes, for example. It can also be identified as the nutrients arising from the quality of the soil it is grown in – the levels of minerals and nutrients in the soil itself. This is a complex relationship involving many dimensions to the creation of the food itself and rarely noted on any sort of food packaging. The general rule of thumb is that foods grown in an organic or sustainable culture are denser in nutrients than other products.

The following table demonstrates some of the nutrient breakdowns of the appropriate foods for you to consume.

Example	Average Serving	Calorie content	Nutrient content
Brussels sprouts	250g	28	Vitamins A, C, K; fiber; calcium; and folate
Cantaloupe	500g, cut	54	Calcium; magnesium; potassium.

	into small pieces		Vitamins include A, C, and K; a variety of antioxidants
Kale	500g	8	Disease inhibiting nutrients. Vitamins A, C, K; fiber; and plant-based omega-3 fatty acids
Quinoa	250g, cooked	111	A protein rich in fiber, iron, zinc. Vitamin B, magnesium, potassium, and calcium
Salmon	3 oz.	144	Great protein source, magnesium, potassium, selenium. Vitamin B12, D, and omega-3 fatty acids
Sweet potato	1 med	115	Potassium. Vitamin A, B6, C. Good source of beta-carotene, which is an antioxidant that inhibits free radicals
Walnuts	125g, medium chopped	191	High in omega-3 fatty acids, protein, iron, potassium, zinc, and unsaturated fats. These help with the absorption of vitamins A, D, E, K.

Below, you will find a general overview of food groupings and recommended choices within each group. Each selection is recognized as nutrient-rich and suitable for your healthy living diet plan. Remember to follow the meal size listed above, with your physician recommended vitamin supplements, and you will be on the right path to a quality enriched life.

Grains

Grains are a lovely source of fiber and what are known as complex carbohydrates. These foods assist you in feeling full for more extended periods, give you more sustained energy, and also help you not to overeat. Make sure you check the packaging for the essential words 'whole grains' and must at least contain 3 grams of fiber for each serving.

Some recommended examples of grains are steel cut oats, rolled oats, any product made with 100% whole wheat, wheat, multi-grain crackers, brown and wild rice only, and other grains including barley, quinoa, corn (whole), and buckwheat.

Meat

There is an abundance of lean cuts of meat on the market today. Take your time to search for the keywords "loin, leg, or round" in the cut. Be sure to trim off all fat before cooking. The healthiest way to prepare your choice is to broil, bake, or roast. Try to limit your consumption of lamb, veal, pork, and beef as these meats, even though they may be a lean cut, contain a higher source of fat than other protein choices.

Recommended choices are ground turkey, chicken breast, lean cuts of steak, beef, pork, lamb, and veal.

Fish and Seafood

Choose only fresh fish which has a clean smell, and the flesh is of a firm consistency. If you do not have access to fresh fish, you can select frozen or canned with low-salt only. Fish that are caught in the wild are the best source of omega 3's. Poach, steam bake or broil your selection for the healthiest eating choices.

Recommended selections of fish and seafood include salmon,

white fish, tuna, scallops, shrimp, mussels, and lobster (without any additional fat added).

Non-meat sources of protein also can be nutrient-rich such as all beans, peanut butter, nut butter, seeds (dry roasted, unsalted, or raw), lentils, chickpeas, milk alternatives such as soy, almond, or rice.

Dairy foods

Make sure always to choose low-fat or skim milk options. Replace your coffee cream with evaporated skim milk and look for the fat-free cheeses. These will generally consist of the older, harder cheeses. Some dairy foods are ricotta made from skim milk, cottage cheese – low fat only, plain yogurt, non-fat.

Fruits and Vegetables

Naturally low in fat, these will add much-needed nutrients and variety to your diet. Look for colorful varieties. The richer the color, the higher the nutrient value. Organic produce is pesticide-free and tends to have a higher nutrient value than non-organic choices.

Examples are kale, spinach, swiss chard, broccoli, cauliflower, asparagus, avocados, yams, turnips, parsnips, carrots, pumpkins, sweet potato, squash, peas, green beans, bell peppers, cabbage, bok choy, romaine lettuce, brussel sprouts, tomatoes, apples, mangos, berries, cherries, bananas, pineapple, papaya, plums, grapes, citrus fruits, peaches, melons, pears.

A good rule of thumb is that the primary source of your nutrient-rich foods is in the perimeter or outer circle of your grocery store. Normally, the further in you go to any large chain food store, the more processed the food is. Try organic grocers or even Farmers Markets for the best source of locally grown produce. They tend to be slightly cheaper and of higher nutritional quality than the products brought in by large supermarkets. Plus, you get to know your food suppliers, creating a connection to your food that you might not have enjoyed previously.

Chapter 4: Two-week meal plan

Waking up in the morning to a pre-determined plan of action can be both encouraging and daunting. Knowing what you have meticulously written out the night (or week) before may not be what you feel like at the moment. The five-day meal plan listed below is a suggestion of how to create one that contains variety and balance.

This does not suggest that you will have to follow a pre-determined plan of what to eat every day for the rest of your life. The formation of a healthy lifestyle is largely based on the creation of healthy habits. These habits must be practiced for a significant amount of time, one to three years before they become an unconscious part of who you are. What I'm suggesting here is that you have to re-train yourself to make healthy food and lifestyle choices. This will require constant awareness on your part. One way to help this awareness is on those days when you just want 'one teeny-weeny little break' in training, is a plan of action. Something you can look at, sigh, and acknowledge that this is the choice you want to make and get on with it.

Meal plans not only bolster our re-training regime, but they also provide us an opportunity to seek out new recipe options, try foods we may never have before, and allow us to practice some creativity with flavor compositions for our dining choices. It also gives you the chance to see what ingredients you will need for the week ahead, allowing you to stock your kitchen with the food you want to eat rather than grabbing whatever comes to hand in the grocery store. This is a much better approach. Failing to prepare is preparing to fail.

Be sensitive that for this diet plan to work, you have to enjoy what you are eating. I can guarantee that if you are eating foods that you feel you have to eat (say an eggplant chard smoothie), you will not experience lasting success. It is far better to experiment with the food choices you have available to you, playing with the recipes like spices and ingredients. For example, substitute broccoli instead of brussel sprouts, thus creating food you are excited about eating. You will be sure to stay on track with your goals if you allow yourself this freedom.

Further to this is that with your new diet choices, you might discover that you will need to purchase in smaller quantities. Fresh fruits and vegetables tend to last about a week in the fridge before they go in strange colors, limp, and overall uneatable. Purchasing only enough for the week (besides the extra snack options) will mean you are eating the freshest food possible. Unless, of course, you have a farm market stand, you can visit every day. Not only does this mean you are consuming the freshest produce, but it also requires you to move more to go out and get it. Double bonus in the overall life plan.

What follows is an example of a two-week meal plan once all of your restrictions have been removed, and your primary goal is maintaining your success.

Day 1
Breakfast: Lettuce Power Pack
Snack: Orange is the New Green Smoothie (if needed)
Lunch: Cowboy Caesar
Dinner: Taj Mahal Salad
Dessert: Citrus fruit cup – pieces of mango, pineapple and orange with a dollop of fat-free yogurt (if needed)

Day 2
Breakfast: Sunday Morning Special
Snack: Hulk's Jade Drink (if needed)
Lunch: Frank Sinatra Soup

| Supper: | Rainbow Fillet Almandine |
| Dessert: | Peanut Butter Cookie (if needed) |

Day 3

Breakfast:	Luscious Lip-Smacking Smoothie
Snack;	Greek Egg Muffin (if needed)
Lunch:	Taj Mahal Salad
Dinner:	Amazon Pork Stew
Dessert:	Almond Chocolate Mousse (if needed)

Day 4

Breakfast:	Scrambled Eggs
Snack:	Easy and Light Salad (if needed)
Lunch:	Ham and Bean Soup
Dinner:	Beef Ginger Stir Fry
Dessert:	Rhubarb Apple Popsicle (if needed)

Day 5

Breakfast:	Greek Egg Muffin
Snack:	Rain Forest Smoothie (if needed)
Lunch:	Amazon Beef Stew
Dinner:	Orange Fidelity Soup
Dessert:	Bella's Apple Crisp (if needed)

Day 6

Breakfast:	Rain Forest Smoothie
Snack:	Red Energy Wonders
Lunch:	Re-fried Beans with a Twist
Dinner:	Ham & Bean Soup

Dessert: Peanut Butter Joy Cookies (if needed)

Day 7
Breakfast: Simple Sunshine Scramble
Snack: Luscious Lip Smacking Smoothie (if needed)
Lunch: Ginger Beef Veggie Stir Fry
Dinner: Frank Sinatra Soup
Dessert: Chocolate Almond Ginger Mousse (if needed)

Day 8
Breakfast: Lettuce Power Pack
Snack: Orange is the New Green Smoothie (if needed)
Lunch: Cowboy Caesar
Dinner: Taj Mahal Salad
Dessert: Citrus fruit cup – pieces of mango, pineapple and
orange with a dollop of fat-free yogurt (if needed)

Day 9
Breakfast: Sunday Morning Special
Snack: Hulk's Jade Drink (if needed)
Lunch: Frank Sinatra Soup
Supper: Rainbow Fillet Almandine
Dessert: Peanut Butter Cookie (if needed)

Day 10
Breakfast: Luscious Lip-Smacking Smoothie
Snack;   Greek Egg Muffin (if needed)
Lunch: Taj Mahal Salad
Dinner: Amazon Pork Stew
Dessert: Almond Chocolate Mousse (if needed)

Day 11

Breakfast:	Scrambled Eggs
Snack:	Easy and Light Salad (if needed)
Lunch:	Ham and Bean Soup
Dinner:	Beef Ginger Stir Fry
Dessert:	Rhubarb Apple Popsicle (if needed)

Day 12

Breakfast:	Greek Egg Muffin
Snack:	Rain Forest Smoothie (if needed)
Lunch:	Amazon Beef Stew
Dinner:	Orange Fidelity Soup
Dessert:	Bella's Apple Crisp (if needed)

Day 13

Breakfast:	Rain Forest Smoothie
Snack:	Red Energy Wonders
Lunch:	Re-fried Beans with a Twist
Dinner:	Ham & Bean Soup
Dessert:	Peanut Butter Joy Cookies (if needed)

Day 14

Breakfast:	Simple Sunshine Scramble
Snack:	Luscious Lip-Smacking Smoothie (if needed)
Lunch:	Ginger Beef Veggie Stir Fry
Dinner:	Frank Sinatra Soup
Dessert:	Chocolate Almond Ginger Mousse (if needed)

Chapter 5: Recipes That Nourish and Delight

Broth

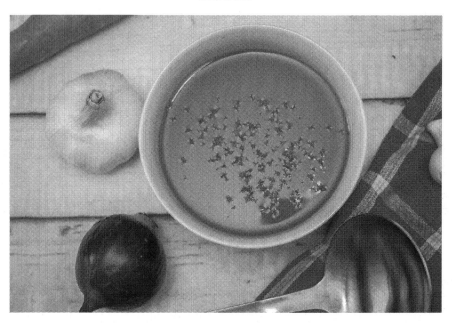

Vibrant Veggie Broth

Ingredients:

- 2 leeks, roughly chopped
- 3 sticks celery, roughly chopped
- 1 onion, large roughly chopped
- 2 cloves garlic, unpeeled, unchopped
- 1 pepper, yellow, seeded, and chopped
- 1 parsnip, chopped
- 4 large mushrooms (whole)
- 1 medium tomato, roughly chopped
- 3 bay leaves, dried

- a handful of parsley, fresh
- 3 sprigs of thyme, fresh
- 1 sprig of rosemary, fresh
- 1 teaspoon salt
- 8 whole black peppercorns
- 3 liters of cold water

Procedure:

1. Put all of your washed and chopped ingredients into a large soup pot with the water.
2. Bring to a boil, turn down the heat, and let the soup simmer for thirty minutes, stirring occasionally.
3. Let the soup cool down, then strain off and discard all of the vegetables. You can freeze this stock in batches, using it as needed.

Soothing Chicken Broth

Ingredients:

- 1 whole chicken approx. 1.3 kg
- 6stalks of celery, roughly chopped
- 6 carrots, large, roughly chopped
- 1 leek, trimmed and chopped
- 1 onion, brown and chopped
- 4 stems of fresh parsley
- 2 bay leaves, dried
- 10 – 15 whole black peppercorns
- 1/2 teaspoon salt
- 3 liters of cold water

Procedure:

1. Put the whole chicken into a large soup pot. Gently pour the water over the top. Cover the pot and bring the water to a boil. Remove any scum that might be floating on the surface (a soup spoon works well for this) during the cooking process.
2. Uncover the pot and add all of the other prepped ingredients. Turn the heat down to a medium and allow to cook, uncovered, for about one and a half hours. Keep an eye out for scum and remove as needed.
3. Using a pair of tongs remove the chicken from the soup broth. You can choose to discard the chicken or puree it for inclusion with other meals. Allow the chicken to cool before removing the meat from the bones and pureeing it with a bit of the stock added for flavor and juiciness.
4. Taste the broth and adjust the seasoning. Remember to keep it fairly mild/bland if you are using this for the first week or two

after surgery. Allow the broth to cool overnight in the fridge. You can skim any accumulated fat off of the top of the cold soup in the morning.

Broiled Beef Broth

Ingredients:

- 2 kilograms soup bones (beef shanks)
- 3 carrots, medium,   roughly chopped
- 3 celery stalks, roughly chopped
- 2 onions, medium,   roughly chopped
- 150 ml warm water (approx. 47C degrees)
- 3bay leaves, dried
- 3 cloves garlic
- 10 black peppercorns, whole
- 4 sprigs parsley, fresh
- 1 tsp. thyme, dried
- 1 tsp. marjoram, dried
- 1 tsp. oregano, dried
- cold water

Procedure:

1. Preheat the oven to 235 degrees. Place the soup pans in a large roasting pan and bake for thirty minutes, uncovered. Add in the vegetables and continue to bake for another thirty minutes. Drain any fat.
2. With a slotted spoon, transfer your ingredients into a large Dutch oven. Place the warmed water in the roasting pan and swirl it around to dislodge the browned bits. Pour this over the ingredients in the Dutch oven. Add the remaining ingredients and plenty of cold water, just covering the contents. Bring to a boil, lower the heat, letting the soup simmer for about five hours uncovered. Skim the foam off and add additional water if required during the first two hours to keep the ingredients

covered.

3. Turn the heat off and remove the bones from the pot. You can save the meat for another use, discarding the bones. Allow the broth to cool slightly before straining through a cheese-cloth placed over a colander. Discard the vegetables and herbs. Skim the fat if you are using the broth right away. You can also refrigerate the broth overnight and skim the fat from the top in the morning.

4. The broth can be stored in the fridge for three days or frozen.

Bone Broth

Ingredients:

- 1 or 2 ltr Water
- 1/2 or 1 lb Bones
- 4 cloves of Garlic
- 1 sliced Carrot
- 1/4th Onion (sliced)
- 1 stalk of Celery (sliced)
- 1 teaspoon Black peppercorns (whole)
- 1 pinch Red pepper (crushed)
- Sea salt according to taste

Procedure:

1. Place all the ingredients in one big slow cooker. Put it on low heat and simmer the broth for a minimum of 48 hours.
2. Add water if needed to make up for the evaporation.
3. Use a sieve or fine cloth to strain the broth and separate the solids.
4. Keep it in the fridge for 4 days. Otherwise, you can freeze it for 3 months.
5. You can warm it or drink it chilled. Or else, add it to any recipe of your choice.

Turkey Gravy

Ingredients:

- 2 tbsp fresh Sage (chopped finely)
- 4 cups or 32 oz Turkey stock (unsalted)
- 2 tbsp fresh Thyme (chopped finely)
- 1 cup or 8 oz skimmed Milk
- 1/4th cup of Cornstarch

Procedure:

1. After roasting the turkey put the pan on medium heat. Put two cups of the turkey stock in the pan. Cook and stir for 5 minutes till the browned bits and drippings dissolve. Put a strainer on one fat separator vessel. Then pour the pan drippings on it. Add sufficient stock to this so that you can make 4 cups.
2. In case, you do not have one fat separator vessel put some ice cubes in the liquid. Then refrigerate it for ten minutes. Remove the hardened fat and put the stock in a saucepan. The liquid should be equal to 4 cups. Place the pan on medium heat. Simmer the stock. Add thyme and sage. Keep simmering until the quantity of stock reduces to 3 cups.
3. Pour milk in one small bowl. Put cornstarch in it and mix evenly. Then pour this mixture in the stock. Stir slowly. Cook till it starts boiling. Keep stirring till the stock thickens. This may take 3 or 5 minutes.
4. Transfer it to a warm gravy boat for serving.

Smoothies

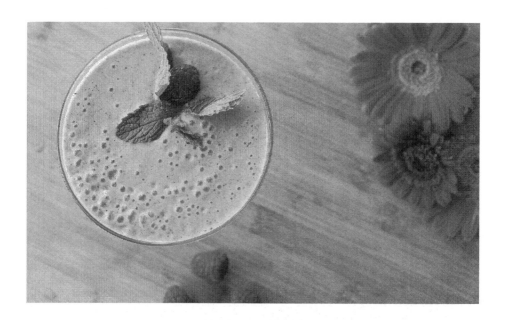

You can prepare single serving smoothies in advance. Simply make the recipe and freeze in the portion size you require. Take a portion out of the freezer twenty minutes before serving, letting it stand at room temperature. Take care to stir several times during the thawing process.

Rain Forest Smoothie

Ingredients:

- 115 ml Greek yogurt, plain, non-fat
- 225 g fresh, baby spinach leaves
- 250 ml banana slices, frozen (one medium)
- 125 ml chunks of frozen pineapple
- 3 teaspoons chia seeds
- 125 ml almond (or rice) milk, unsweetened

Procedure:

1. Place all ingredients in the blender, wet ones first, and whirl well. Add water or more almond milk for a more fluid consistency.

Hulk's Jade Drink

Ingredients:

- 625 ml kale leaves, stems removed
- 250 ml pineapple, cut in cubes
- 75 ml unsweetened apple juice
- 75 ml of water
- 125 ml green grapes, seedless and frozen
- 125 ml apple chopped, preferably Granny Smith

Procedure:

1. Place all of the ingredients in the blender, wet ones first, and whirl for three minutes. Chill for one to two hours if preparing in advance. Be sure to stir before serving.

Orange is the New Green

Ingredients:

- 250 ml almond (or rice) milk, unsweetened, vanilla flavor
- 125 ml butternut squash cooked and cut into cubes, frozen
- 1/2 tsp cinnamon, ground or 1/8 tsp nutmeg, ground
- 1 serving protein powder

Procedure:

1. Place the ingredients into the blender, wet ones first, and whirl for two minutes. You can add 125 ml of baby green spinach leaves for extra nutrients if you want.

Luscious Lip-Smacking Smoothie

This is one balanced liquid treat! This contains a bit of everything you need in one glass, vegetables, fruit, the good kind of fats, fiber, and protein. Enjoy!

Ingredients:

- 250 ml unsweetened almond milk
- 1 banana, small, cut into chunks and frozen
- 1 tbsp nut butter – almond or peanut
- 1 half of a small, ripe avocado
- 125 ml raw baby spinach leaves
- 1 serving protein powder

Procedure:

1. Place all ingredients in the blender, wet ones first, whirl for two minutes and enjoy.

Basic Smoothie

Ingredients:

- Half a cup of plain Yogurt
- One cup of fresh fruit (any fruit of choice)
- One tablespoon sweetener (such as Truvia or Splenda)
- One cup Almond Milk (without sugar)

Procedure:

1. Put the yogurt, fruit, sweetener, and almond milk in a blender.
2. Pulse for some seconds, repeat it a few times till the mixture becomes smooth.
3. Add some ice. Blend once again. Enjoy a healthy and delicious smoothie.

Delicious Lemon and Blueberry Smoothie

Ingredients:

- 3 cups of fresh Spinach
- Half a cup of fresh Coriander
- 2 cups of Water
- 1 Lemon
- 2 cups of Blueberries
- 1" fresh Ginger

Procedure:

1. Place all ingredients in the blender, wet ones first, whirl for two minutes and enjoy.

Refreshing Watermelon Smoothie

Ingredients:

- One and a half cups of Watermelon chunks (no seeds)
- One and a half cups of Strawberries (frozen)
- 2 tbsp Lime juice
- 3 leaves of Mint

- Half a cup of Water
- 1 cup of Ice

Procedure:

1. Place all ingredients in the blender, wet ones first, whirl for two minutes and enjoy.

Tasty Tropical Smoothie

Ingredients:

- 2 cups of Blueberries
- 3 cups of Veggies
- 1 cup of canned Coconut milk
- Half a cup of Water
- 1 tsp of Vanilla extract
- 1 handful Ice
- 1 scoop of Protein powder

Procedure:

1. Place all ingredients in the blender, wet ones first, whirl for two minutes and enjoy.

Yummy Avocado and Mint Smoothie

Ingredients:

- One and a half cups of Blueberries
- One and a half cups of seeded Avocado
- One and a half cups of Coconut water
- 4 to 6 Mint leaves
- 1 tbsp Lime juice
- Half a cup of Water

Procedure:

1. Place all ingredients in the blender, wet ones first, whirl for two minutes and enjoy.

Classic Smoothie

Ingredients:

- 1 cup of Strawberries
- 3 cups of Kale
- 1 cup of Raspberries
- 1/4th cup of fresh Parsley
- Half a cup of Coconut water
- 1 tbsp Lemon juice
- 1 cup of Ice
- Half a cup of Water

Procedure:

1. Place all ingredients in the blender, wet ones first, whirl for two minutes and enjoy.

Breakfast Time

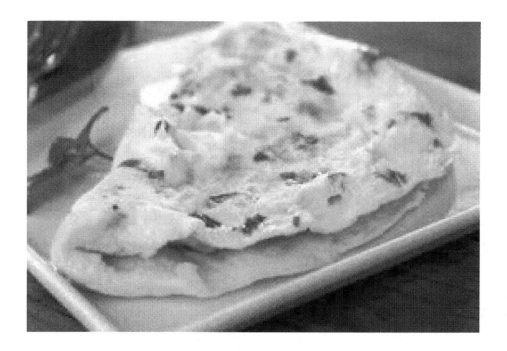

Be sure never to skip this most important meal of the day. Nourish and fortify yourself for the adventures ahead!

Lettuce Power Pack

Makes one serving.

Ingredients:

- 1 egg, large
- 1 white of an egg, large
- 125 ml baby spinach leaves, small pieces
- 2 tbsp fat-free feta, crumbled
- 2 tomato, Roma, small pieces

- pinch of salt, kosher or sea
- black pepper
- 1 large lettuce leaf, preferably not iceberg

Procedure:

1. Place the first seven ingredients in a bowl and whisk well. Have a nonstick pan heating on medium heat, add the combined mixture, and cook to the consistency of your choice. Place the cooked ingredients on one end of the leaf and roll up.

Greek Egg Muffins

Makes six servings.
Can be made ahead and enjoyed throughout the week for breakfast or lunch.

Ingredients:

- 5 eggs large
- 10 cherry tomatoes, quartered
- 5 artichoke hearts, marinated and diced
- 125 ml mozzarella cheese, low-fat and shredded
- 2 tbsp basil, fresh and minced
- pepper and salt for taste
- cooking spray for the muffin tin

Procedure:

1. While the oven is preheating to 350 degrees, break the eggs into a bowl and whisk well until smooth.
2. Combine the rest of the ingredients to the eggs and stir gently together.
3. Coat the muffin tin cups lightly with the cooking spray.
4. Spoon the egg mixture into six cups, dividing it equally.
5. Bake for twenty minutes or 'til the eggs is set.
6. Let cool for a minute before savoring or store in the fridge to be enjoyed later.

Sunday Morning Special

Makes one serving.

You can start to enjoy these about six weeks after your surgery. This single serving recipe can be eaten at any time of day, any day of the week. Try replacing the savory ingredients with two tablespoons of Splenda for a more traditional pancake taste.

Ingredients:

- 125 ml cottage cheese, low fat
- 1 egg, large
- 75 ml onion   diced
- 1/4 tsp garlic   minced
- 1 generous tbsp whole wheat flour
- pepper and salt for taste
- cooking spray for the pan

Procedure:

1. Spray the pan and pre-heat for a minute.
2. Sauté the garlic and onions, while stirring together the egg, cottage cheese, flour and pepper, and salt.
3. Add the cooked ingredients to the bowl mixture, stirring until well-combined.
4. Spray the pan again and spoon in the mixture to pan. Create 4 pancakes.
5. Cook on each side for four minutes.

Simple Sunshine Scramble

Makes one serving.

Ingredients:

- 1 egg
- 1 clove garlic, small   minced
- 1 tsp pesto
- 2 cherry tomatoes, quartered
- 1 piece bacon turkey, crumbled
- 1 tsp parmesan cheese, grated fine
- cooking spray for the pan

Procedure:

1. Lightly whisk the egg in a mixing bowl. Add a dash of water to the egg and the pesto. Whisk again lightly.
2. Spray the pan lightly with cooking spray and heat to medium-high.
3. Sauté the garlic until the aroma is released. Stir in bacon to crisp.
4. Slide pan contents out onto a side dish. Add tomatoes to the pan, sauté until liquid is almost gone.
5. Add egg mixture to the pan and cook as for how you prefer your scrambled eggs. Stir in the bacon/garlic mixture and parmesan cheese just before the eggs are cooked.
6. Serve with a slice of orange for that complete sunshine feel.

Black Beans Puree with Scrambled Eggs

Ingredients:

- For making the scrambled egg part of the recipe
- 1/8 teaspoon Salt
- 1 egg
- 1/8 teaspoon pepper
- Black beans puree
- 3 tablespoons Enchilada sauce (green)
- 1/2 cup rinsed Black beans
- 2 tablespoon Vegetable or chicken broth
- 1 tablespoon protein powder

Procedure:

Black beans puree:
1. Put the beans in some small sized saucepan on medium heat. Then put the enchilada sauce. Heat for 2 minutes. Keep stirring all the time. Then add the chicken broth.
2. Shift the mixture to one blender or use one hand blender to make a smooth mixture. Transfer it into one bowl.
3. Let it cool a bit and then mix the protein powder. Stir well. Cover it to keep it warm till you cook the egg.
4. Keep the leftovers in the fridge so that you can eat them at some other time.

Scrambled egg:
1. Heat one non-stick pan on medium heat. In the meantime, put the egg in one small bowl and whisk it well to incorporate air into it.
2. Pour the egg into the heated pan. Sprinkle pepper and salt. Use one rubber spatula for moving the egg in the pan while it is getting cooked. When it is almost done and still has a slightly liquid texture, you should fold it and take it out on a plate.
3. Put 1 tablespoon of the black beans puree. Also, put 1 teaspoon

of enchilada sauce (green).
4. Note: This recipe is for making 1 serving. It provides approximately 5 grams of fat, 11 grams of proteins, and 6 grams of carbohydrates.

Ricotta Baked in the Oven

Ingredients:

- 1/4th cup Parmesan cheese (grated)
- 1/2 cup Ricotta cheese (low fat)
- 1 teaspoon Dijon mustard
- 1 teaspoon Thyme (ground)
- 1/4th cup Cheddar cheese (shredded)
- 1 egg

Procedure:

1. Heat the oven to a temperature of 400F.
2. Put all the ingredients in one bowl. Stir and mix them well. The mixture will appear to be gritty and slightly brown. But it must be smooth.
3. Use one cookie scoop and divide the mixture into 4 wells of the muffin pan. You can use muffin pans made of silicone as you can use them easily and clean them quickly.
4. Bake it for about 20 minutes. Then remove from the oven and let it cool a bit. It is ready to be served.
5. Note: This recipe is for making four ricotta muffins. Every muffin provides approximately 4 grams of fat, 4 grams of carbohydrates and 8 grams of proteins

Poached Eggs Italian Style

Ingredients:

- 3 to 4 pieces of jarred Red pepper (roasted and sliced)
- 16 oz of Marinara sauce (with the lowest level of sugar)
- 4 eggs
- 4 leaves of fresh basil
- 1 pinch of salt
- 1 pinch of pepper

Procedure:

1. Heat a big, rimmed skillet on medium heat.
2. Put the marinara sauce. Then add the red peppers.
3. Crack the eggs one by one making a "well" with the back of one spoon.
4. Sprinkle pepper and salt.
5. Allow it to cook till the eggs become firm or for around 12 minutes. If you'd like you can put the lid for 2 minutes at the end.
6. Remove from the heat. Sprinkle basil and serve in a bowl or plate.
7. Note
8. Every serving provides approximately 6 grams of fat, 8 grams of proteins, and 7 grams of carbohydrates.

Crustless Cheesy Quiche

Ingredients:

- 4 oz cubed baby Swiss (low fat)
- 6 oz Chicken breasts (cut into 1-inch cubes and grilled)
- 10 oz shredded Mozzarella cheese (low fat)
- 3 big eggs
- Non-stick cooking spray
- 1 cup Milk (skimmed)
- Oregano for seasoning (optional)

Procedure:

1. Heat the oven beforehand to a temperature of 400 degrees.
2. Spray the non-stick cooking spray on one 9-inch pie pan.
3. Put the chicken and baby Swiss cubes in the pan.
4. Spread Mozzarella cheese on top.
5. Sprinkle oregano on it for taste.
6. Put the skimmed milk and eggs in one separate bowl and whip them. Pour this on the mixture of cheese and chicken.
7. Bake for forty minutes at a temperature of 400 degrees.
8. Serve after it cools down or cover it with a tin foil and refrigerate.
9. You can add cooked green pepper, tomatoes, onions, and other vegetables according to your preference.

Baked Cottage Cheese

Ingredients:

- 2 Eggs
- 2 cups Cottage cheese (fat-free or low-fat)
- 1 (10 oz) pack frozen and thawed Spinach
- Half a cup of Parmesan cheese

Procedure:

1. Heat the oven beforehand to a temperature of 350 degrees.
2. Mix all the ingredients in a big bowl.
3. Put evenly in a pan (8x8).
4. Bake for twenty to thirty minutes.
5. Leave it for 5 minutes and then serve.
6. Season according to taste using salt, garlic, and pepper.

Crispy Tuna Patty

Ingredients:

- 16 thin Crackers (made of wheat, crushed)
- Whites of 4 eggs
- 4 cans of 3 oz Tuna packed in water
- 1/4th cup Carrot (grated)
- 1/4th cup water chestnuts (chopped), red pepper (diced) or capers
- 1 tbsp Onion (minced)
- Pepper, dried mustard and dill, to taste

Procedure:

1. Mix all the ingredients.
2. Use your hands to form 8 patties with the mixture.
3. Spray non-stick cooking spray on one skillet and place it on medium heat.
4. Cook the patties for 2 or 3 minutes on both the sides till they become golden brown.

Orange Roughy Lemon-Broiled

Ingredients:

- 3 tbsp Lemon juice
- 16 oz fillets of Orange Roughy (4 oz each)
- 1/4th tsp Pepper (ground)
- 1 tbsp Olive oil
- 1 tbsp Dijon mustard
- 8 medium-sized Lemon wedges

Procedure:

1. Cover one baking sheet or a rack of one broiler pan with a tin foil. Spray some cooking spray on it.
2. Mix lemon juice, olive oil, ground pepper, and mustard.
3. Place the fillets on the baking sheet or rack.
4. Use half of the lemon mixture to brush the fillets. Reserve the rest of it.
5. Broil the fillets for about 5 minutes.
6. Drizzle the rest of the lemon mixture on the fillets. Add pepper according to taste. Then serve with the lemon wedges.

Fish Fillet Pan-Fried

Ingredients:

- 8 oz Fish fillets
- 1 and 1/3rd tbsp Parsley (chopped)
- 3 tbsp yellow cornmeal
- 1/4th tsp Celery seeds (ground)
- 1/4th tsp Black pepper (ground)
- 1 pinch of Salt
- 2 tsp Olive oil

Procedure:

1. Clean the fish fillets. Remove all the bones.
2. Mix cornmeal, pepper, celery seeds, chopped parsley, and salt.
3. Cover the fish with the cornmeal mixture. Press it on the fish.
4. Heat the oil in one non-stick skillet. Cook each side of the fish for 2 or 3 minutes. The fillets should be crisp and brown. They should flake easily when a fork is pierced.

Turkey Turnovers

Ingredients:

- 1 lb Turkey only breast meat (ground)
- 1 cup shredded Cheese (low-fat)
- 1 packet Onion soup
- 3 tubes Crescent rolls refrigerated (8 in every tube)

Procedure:

1. Heat the oven beforehand to a temperature of 350 degrees.
2. Mix the soup with the meat in a skillet. Cook properly till it becomes brown.
3. Put the cheese.
4. Unroll dough and separate the rolls. Cut every triangle into half.
5. Place a spoonful of the cooked meat in the center of every triangle.
6. Fold then and seal the edges. Put on a cookie sheet.
7. Bake for fifteen minutes.

Whopper Burger

Ingredients:

- One Boca Burger
- 1 Hamburger bun (whole wheat)
- 1 tbsp Miracle Whip
- 1 tbsp Ketchup
- 1 tbsp Mustard
- Tomato
- Lettuce
- Onion

Procedure:

1. Prepare the Boca Burger according to the instructions given on the package.
2. Put the burger on the bun with ketchup, miracle whip, tomato, onion, and lettuce.

Soups

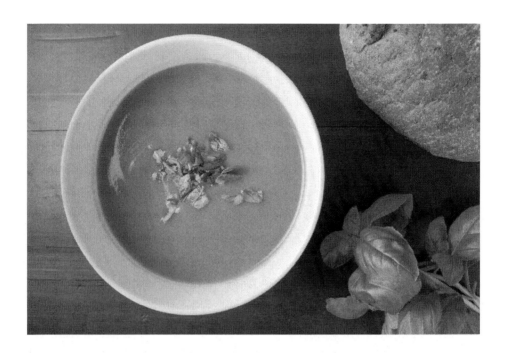

Ham & Bean

Makes ten servings.

Ingredients:

- 125 ml celery, chopped fine
- 125 ml carrots, chopped fine
- 125 ml onion minced
- 1 clove garlic, minced
- 350 ml ham, cubed
- 1/8 tsp pepper, cayenne
- 1/4 tsp cumin, dried
- 1/4 tsp sea salt

- 1 can beans, navy
- 250 ml broth, chicken or veggie
- 250 ml of water

Procedure:

1. Brown ham in a soup pot or large saucepan on medium heat.
2. Pour in water, scraping the glaze off the bottom of the pan.
3. Pour in the broth.
4. Add in the beans. Be sure to drain the liquid from the can and rinse the beans before adding.
5. Add in the remaining ingredients and stir well.
6. Bring soup to a boil, turn heat to simmer, and let it be for one to three hours (the longer it cooks, the better it tastes), stirring occasionally.

Frank Sinatra Soup

Makes ten servings.

Ingredients:

- 1 tbsp olive oil
- 1 onion, diced
- 4cloves garlic, minced
- 250 ml carrots, diced
- 500 ml broccoli florets, chopped into small pieces
- 750 ml cauliflower florets, chopped into small pieces
- 1 1/2 liters of vegetable broth
- 4 tomatoes, medium, diced
- 1 tbsp dried Italian herb mix
- Pinch Red Pepper flakes, crushed, a pinch
- Black pepper and salt for taste
- Parmesan cheese, grated, for sprinkling on top
- Fresh Parsley, chopped, for sprinkling on top

Procedure:

1. Heat the oil in a large soup pot over medium heat.
2. Add the garlic and onion. Cook until fragrant for about two minutes.
3. Stir in the carrot. Continue cooking for another two-three minutes.
4. Pour in the broth, stir in the tomatoes, herbs pinch of red pepper flakes, black pepper, and salt.
5. Bring the ingredients to a boil. Lower the heat and simmer for five minutes.
6. Add in the broccoli and cauliflower, simmering all the while until the vegetables are cooked through but still crunchy.

This may take five minutes.

7. Taste and adjust your seasoning.
8. Serve yourself a bowl, sprinkling the cheese and parsley on top.
9. If you would like to enjoy this as a slightly thicker soup, stir one tbsp of coconut flour or cornstarch into 75 ml of cold water. Add this to the soup and continue to cook for an additional five minutes after the vegetables have finished cooking.

Orange Fidelity

Makes twelve servings.

Ingredients:

- 1 onion, medium and sliced
- 2 pears, small, halved, unpeeled, cored and chopped small
- 3 sprigs thyme
- 2 tbsps. olive oil, Extra Virgin
- 1-kilo butternut squash, halved, seeded, unpeeled
- 250 ml broth, chicken or vegetable
- 500 ml milk, non-fat
- Garnish: 75 ml pecan pieces, toasted or almonds

Procedure:

1. Heat oven to 400°F.
2. On a cookie sheet covered with parchment paper, place the pears, onions & thyme. Sprinkle with the olive oil.
3. On top of this, place the two squash halves.
4. Roast for fifty-sixty minutes. It is done when you can pierce the squash with a fork. Remove from oven and let cool.
5. Scoop the flesh from the squash, discarding the peel.
6. Place squash flesh and pan contents (without the parchment paper) into a blender or food processor. Blend.
7. Pour this into a large soup pot, add the broth, and simmer for ten minutes.
8. Stir in the milk and continue to simmer for another eight minutes.
9. Garnish with the nut pieces and serve.
10. Do not add the pecans as garnish unless you are more than six months post-procedure.

Potato Broccoli Soup

Ingredients:

- Half a cup of Broccoli (chopped)
- 1 cup of Broth
- 1 small sized Potato (chopped)
- 1 tablespoon Corn starch
- Half a cup of Milk
- 2 tablespoons Cheddar cheese (shredded)
- 1 teaspoon Garlic powder
- Pepper and salt according to taste

Procedure:

1. Peel and cut the potato. Then boil it till it becomes soft.
2. Steam the broccoli till it is tender.
3. Put the potato and broccoli in one food processor and make a puree.
4. Mix 1 tablespoon corn starch in 1/4th cup of broth in a saucepan and heat it for one minute till it starts boiling. Slowly add the remaining broth and let it cook till it starts boiling again. The liquid will become thick and creamy because of the corn starch.
5. Put milk, garlic powder, and the puree and stir. Then add the pepper and salt according to taste.
6. Remove it from heat. Put the cheddar cheese and stir till it melts.
7. Serve when it is warm. You can keep the leftovers in the fridge for 3 days.

Black Bean and Pumpkin Soup

Ingredients:

- 2 tbsp Olive oil
- 4 cloves of Garlic (minced)
- 1 medium sized Onion (chopped)
- 1 tbsp Cumin (ground)
- 1 tsp Chilli powder
- 2 cups of Beef broth
- 1/2 tsp Black pepper
- 1 cup diced Tomatoes (canned)
- 2 cans or 15 oz Black beans
- 1 can or 16 oz Pumpkin Puree

Procedure:

1. Heat the oil on medium heat in one soup kettle. Saute garlic, onions, cumin, pepper and chili powder.
2. Stir in the pumpkin, beans, tomatoes, and broth.
3. Simmer uncovered for 25 minutes and occasionally stir till the soup becomes thick.
4. You can serve it as it is or else puree it with one immersion blender and make it smooth.
5. Optional
6. Add Greek yogurt to make it creamier and get more protein.
7. Put 1/2 lb ground meat to get additional proteins.

Mushroom and Wild Rice Soup

Ingredients:

- 1 tbsp Olive oil
- 1/2 white Onion
- 1/4th cup of chopped Carrots
- 1/4th cup of chopped Celery
- One and a half cups of sliced white Mushrooms (fresh)
- Half a cup of white wine
- 2 tbsp flour
- 1/4th tsp dried Thyme
- 1 cup of wild rice (cooked)
- Black pepper
- Two and a half cups of fat-free, low-sodium chicken broth

Procedure:

1. Heat olive oil on medium heat in a stockpot.
2. Put the chopped onions, carrots and celery and cook till they become tender.
3. Add the mushrooms, chicken broth and white wine: cover and cook.
4. Mix the flour, pepper, and thyme in one bowl.
5. Put the wild rice (cooked) in it.
6. Then put this rice mixture in the hot stockpot. Cook on medium heat. Keep stirring till it becomes bubbly and thick.

Tortilla Chicken Soup

Ingredients:

- 2 cups of Black beans salsa
- 1 pound Chicken tenderloins
- 1 teaspoon salt
- 2 teaspoon Mexican spice
- 1 teaspoon ground Cumin
- 4 cups of Water
- 2 cups of frozen Corn
- 4.5-ounce green Chillies
- 10 ounce diced tomatoes
- 2 tablespoons fresh coriander
- 10-ounce black beans
- 1 teaspoon Black pepper
- Cheese and lime juice for garnishing (optional)

Procedure:

1. Rinse the chicken tenderloins. Sprinkle pepper and salt on them before putting them in the crockpot.
2. Put the salsa and the spices. Then cook for 4 hours on low heat.
3. Take out and shred the chicken. Put it back in the crockpot. Add water, additional beans, corn, tomatoes, coriander, and chilies. Cook for 2 more hours.
4. Garnish with cheese and coriander leaves. Add a dash of lime juice and serve.

Taco Soup

Ingredients:

- 1 yellow Onion (small)
- 1 green Pepper (small)
- 1 clove of Garlic
- 1 pound lean Meat (ground)
- 1 teaspoon Cumin
- 1 teaspoon Coriander
- 1 teaspoon Onion powder
- 1 packet of Taco seasoning
- 4-ounce Tomatoes
- Pepper and Salt to taste
- 10-ounce Black beans
- 1 cup prepared salsa
- 2 cup Water or Chicken broth
- Sliced Jalapenos (optional)
- Plain Greek yogurt (optional)
- Shredded Cheese (optional)

Procedure:

1. Mist a pot with some cooking spray. Place it on medium heat. Saute the green pepper and onions for 3 minutes. Then saute garlic for 2 minutes.
2. Put the meat and stir. Drain the meat mixture in case there is excess liquid. Add the taco seasoning.
3. Put the black beans, tomatoes, and salsa. Mix properly. Add water or broth according to the need.
4. Reduce the heat, cover it, and cook till it starts boiling. Turn the heat off. Let it remain covered for some minutes. Then serve in bowls. You can garnish it with sliced jalapenos, Greek yogurt or cheese.

Salads

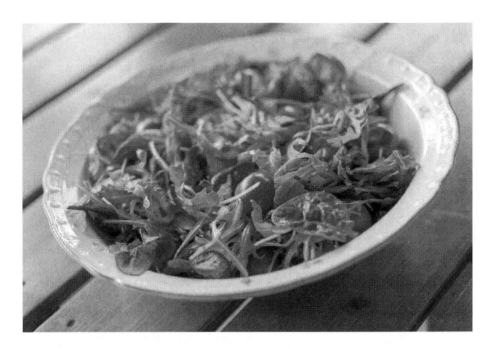

Taj Mahal

Makes 4 servings.

Ingredients:
- 500 ml chicken breast, skinned, de-boned, cooked & cubed
- 1 stalk celery, chopped fine
- 125 ml apple, chopped fine
- 125 ml raisins, let sit in warm water for a few minutes to plump
- 75 ml red onion, chopped fine
- 75 ml cilantro, fresh, roughly chopped
- 75 ml almonds, toasted & sliced
- 125 ml Greek yogurt, plain
- 75 ml mayonnaise, light
- 1 tbsp lime juice, fresh

- 1 tbsp agave syrup or honey
- 1/2 tbsp curry powder, mild
- black pepper and sea salt for taste

Procedure:

1. Drain the raisins. In a large bowl, gently stir them together with the apple, the onions, celery, cilantro, chicken, and almonds.
2. In a smaller bowl, whisk together the yogurt, lime, mayonnaise, syrup, and curry.
3. Pour the dressing over the chicken combination and gently stir to combine.
4. Season with pepper and salt to taste.
5. This salad can be kept in your fridge for up to three days.

Easy and Light

Makes 2 servings.

Ingredients:

- 3 carrots, large, chopped
- 1 zucchini, medium, chopped
- 75 ml basil, fresh, sliced into ribbons
- 400 ml chickpeas, canned, rinsed and drained
- 1 clove garlic, minced
- 1 tomato, large and diced
- 1 tbsp olive oil, Extra virgin
- 1 tbsp green pesto
- Black pepper and salt to taste

Procedure:

1. Gently stir together the vegetables in a large mixing bowl.
2. Whisk the oil, garlic, and pesto, adding more oil or little water to achieve the consistency of the dressing you desire. Note: This can be made an hour before to pack a more potent flavor punch.
3. Pour dressing over the vegetables. Add salt and pepper, tossing together gently.

Thai Inspired Asian Salad

Makes two servings.

Ingredients:

- 1 chicken breast, baked, shredded
- 250 ml cabbage, red, shredded
- 1/2 pepper, bell, cut in thin strips
- 125 ml cilantro, chopped fine
- 75 ml onion, green,   chopped fine
- 125 ml peanuts, chopped very fine
- 75 ml mango, sliced very fine
- Dressing
- 125 ml yogurt, Greek, plain
- 1 tbsp agave or maple syrup
- 1 tbsp lime juice, fresh
- 1/2 tsp tamari sauce
- pinch of red pepper flakes

Procedure:

1. Mix all of the vegetables and chicken in a large bowl until well-combined.
2. Using a fork, combine the dressing ingredients in a measuring cup.
3. Pour dressing over the ingredients and gently toss until everything is well-coated.
4. Serve right away or store in the fridge until you are ready to eat.
5. You can serve this wrapped in a whole grain tortilla or over cold brown rice.

Cowboy Caesar Salad

Makes four servings.

Ingredients:

- 16 oz steak, lean sirloin
- 1 head lettuce, Romaine, washed and chopped
- 1 tomato, large, cut into wedges
- 1 cucumber, chopped
- 1 tbsp parmesan cheese, grated for garnish
- 2 tbsp Caesar dressing, light

Procedure:

1. Preheat grill. Sprinkle both sides of the steak with the pepper and salt. Grill each side for 6 minutes or until desired doneness.
2. Layer four plates with lettuce. Top each serving with tomatoes and cucumbers.
3. Thinly slice the steak against the grain and place equally on top of the lettuce.
4. Drizzle each serving with the Caesar dressing and sprinkle the parmesan on top.

Savvy Spinach Salad

Makes one serving.

Ingredients:

- 250 ml baby spinach, torn into pieces
- 75 ml cucumber, chopped small
- 75 ml apple, chopped small
- 75 ml avocado, chopped
- 1 radish, chopped fine
- 75 ml raisins, let soak in warm water for a couple of minutes before adding then drain
- 75 ml walnuts or pecans, chopped fine
- 1 tbsp feta cheese, crumbled
- 1 tsp basil, fresh and chopped
- 1/2 tbsp olive oil, Extra Virgin

Procedure:

1. Arrange spinach on a plate. Sprinkle the ingredients on in order of listing, so basil is the last item added.
2. Drizzle with the olive oil.

Beans and Salsa Pureed

Makes 4 servings

Ingredients:

- 2 tablespoons Salsa
- 1 can or 15 oz Pinto beans
- 1 scoop Protein powder (unflavored whey)
- 2 tablespoons Chicken broth

Procedure:

1. Mix all the ingredients in one small pan. Place it over medium heat.
2. Stir a few times and let it become warm throughout. Then transfer it to one blender.
3. Blend it at high speed for a few minutes till the mixture becomes smooth. Transfer it to a serving dish.
4. Note: Every serving provides approximately 1 gram of fat, 11 grams of proteins, and 15 grams of carbohydrates.

Chicken Salad Mexican Style

Makes two servings.

Ingredients:

- 1 tablespoon Mayonnaise
- 1 cup Chicken drained (canned)
- 2 teaspoons juice from Salsa (jarred, no chunks)
- 1 teaspoon Taco seasoning

Procedure:

1. Put the canned chicken in a bowl. Break it into small pieces using a fork. Add the mayonnaise and stir well till it is combined properly and becomes soft.
2. Mix the salsa juice and taco seasoning. Serve.
3. Note: Every serving provides approximately 4 grams of fat, 18 grams of proteins, and 2 grams of carbohydrates.

Crab Salad

Makes 1 serving.

Ingredients:

- 1 tablespoon light Mayonnaise
- 2 oz crab (imitation)
- Half a scoop of protein powder (unflavored)
- 1 pinch dried Dill
- 1 pinch of Seafood seasoning

Procedure:

1. Dice the crab meat into small pieces.
2. Mix the light mayonnaise and protein powder until everything is combined properly.
3. Add the seasoning and adjust the taste.
4. Note: It provides approximately 4 grams of fat, 12 grams of proteins, and 8 grams of carbohydrates.

Stuffed Tomatoes and Tuna Salad

Makes 2 servings.

Ingredients:

- 1 can or 4 oz water-packed Tuna (drained)
- 2 Roma tomatoes
- 1/3rd cup Greek yogurt (fat-free)
- 1/4 teaspoon Salt
- 1/4 teaspoon Pepper
- 2 ribs diced Celery
- 1/8 teaspoon Curry powder

Procedure:

1. Cut the tomatoes into halves and remove the seeds.
2. Mix all the ingredients and stuff into the tomato bowls.
3. Note: Every serving provides approximately 1 gram of fat, 15 grams of proteins, and 5 grams of carbohydrates.

Simple Tuna Salad

Ingredients:

- 1 tablespoon Mayonnaise (fat-free)
- 3 oz water-packed Tuna (drained)
- 2 teaspoon Pickle juice
- 1/4 teaspoon Black pepper

Procedure:
1. Drain the tuna and mash it with a fork.
2. Then add the other ingredients. Stir till everything is combined properly.
3. If you want a soft consistency, you can add mayonnaise or pickle juice.

Tuna Salad Tuscan Style

Ingredients:

- 1/4th cup Italian dressing (fat-free)
- 2 cans of water packed Tuna (drained)
- 2 tablespoons Red onion (chopped)
- 2 tablespoons fresh Parsley (chopped)
- 2 tablespoons chopped Red pepper (roasted)
- Zest of 1 Lemon
- 2 cloves of Garlic (minced or pressed)
- Tomato slices (optional)

Procedure:

1. Combine all the ingredients except tomato slices. To make it more interesting, you can scoop the tuna salad on tomato slices.
2. Note: Every serving provides approximately 1 gram of fat, 11 grams of proteins, and 6 grams of carbohydrates.

Chicken Salad with Buffalo Sauce

Ingredients:

- 1/4 cup Mayonnaise (light)
- 2 cups shredded Chicken breast (seasoned with pepper and salt)
- 1/2 teaspoon onion powder
- 5 stalks of Celery
- 3 tablespoons Buffalo sauce

Procedure:

1. Mix all the items and season according to your taste.
2. Note: Every serving provides approximately 3 grams of fat, 17 grams of proteins, and 1 gram of carbohydrates.

Chicken Salad Thai Style

Ingredients:

- 2 stalks of Lemongrass (only the lower 6 inches, thinly sliced)
- 2 cups of Broth, Vegetable stock or Chicken stock (reduced-sodium)
- 1/2" piece of fresh Ginger
- 3 Green onions, 1 halved lengthwise and 2 thinly sliced
- 2 tbsp Lime juice (fresh)
- 3 sprigs of fresh coriander and 3 tbsp chopped coriander
- 2 tbsp Rice vinegar
- 1 and 1/4 lb Chicken breasts
- 1 tbsp Peanut butter
- 1 tbsp minced Shallot
- 1 tbsp Soy sauce (reduced-sodium)
- 1 tbsp Fish sauce
- 1 clove of Garlic
- 3 tbsp Olive oil (extra-virgin)
- 1/2 Green cabbage
- Half a bunch of Spinach
- 1 big Carrot (thinly sliced)
- 1 tbsp unsalted peanuts (dry-roasted and crushed)

Procedure:

1. Combine the lemongrass, coriander sprigs, ginger, stock, and green onion (halved)
   in a big saucepan. Place the pan on high heat and decrease the heat when it is about
   to boil. Simmer for five minutes. Put the chicken and increase the heat so that it
   starts boiling. Again, decrease the heat and simmer for about 3 minutes. Then remove

the pan from heat. Cover it for 5 minutes. Then uncover it and let it cool. When it is sufficiently cool, take out the chicken and keep the stock aside. Shred it into 2" long and 1/2" thick strips. Cover and put it in the fridge.

2. Strain the stock and remove the solids. Put one and a half cups of stock in the

   saucepan. Place it on medium to high heat. Cook for 5 or 6 minutes till it is reduced to half a cup. Let it cool.

3. Put vinegar, lime juice, shallot, fish sauce, shallot, soy sauce, peanut butter, reduced stock and garlic in one blender. Blend till it becomes smooth. Add olive oil slowly while the motor is running. The dressing may be a little thin. Keep it aside.

4. Remove the core of the cabbage and the stems of spinach. Stack their leaves

   separately. Cut them crosswise and make 1/4" strips.

5. Put spinach, shredded chicken, cabbage, carrot, green onions (sliced) and chopped coriander in a big bowl. Pour half portion of dressing on the salad. Then serve the salad equally in separate plates. Use peanuts to garnish it. Place the rest of the dressing on the table.

Protein-Rich Pesto

Ingredients:

- Half a cup of Water
- 1 packet of 10 oz frozen Spinach (chopped)
- 1/3rd cup Cottage cheese
- 2 tbsp Parmesan cheese (grated)
- 1/3rd cup of fresh Basil otherwise 1 tbsp of dried basil
- 2 cloves of Garlic (minced)
- 1 tbsp Olive oil

Procedure:

1. Combine all the ingredients in a food processor or blender.
2. Process or blend till they become smooth.
3. Put half a spoon of the mixture on fish or poultry.

Lunch and Dinner Options

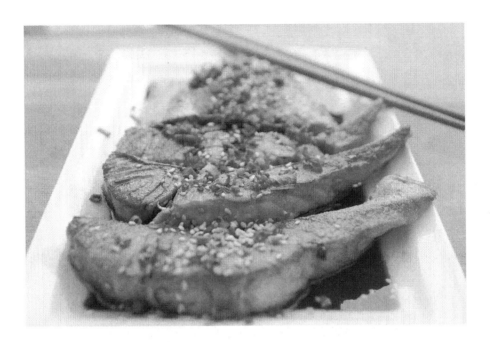

Amazon Pork Stew

Makes four servings.

Ingredients:

- 2 tsp olive oil, Extra virgin
- 1 lb. pork loin, visible fat trimmed off, cut in one-inch cubes
- 325 ml onion, chopped
- 3 garlic cloves
- 2 chipotle peppers canned in adobo sauce, minced
- 1 tsp adobo sauce
- 1 tsp cumin, dried
- 1 Goya Sazon seasoning packet with annatto & coriander or similar

- 500ml chicken broth, no salt added
- 500ml canned tomatoes in juice, no salt added, diced
- 500 ml black beans, no salt added, drained and rinsed
- 1 tsp red pepper flakes, crushed (optional)

Procedure:

1. Heat the oil in a large pot over medium heat.
2. Stir in pork cubes, occasionally stirring for six minutes until brown on all sides.
3. Stir in garlic and onion. Cook for another three minutes until they start to soften.
4. Mix in chipotle, adobo sauce, cumin, and seasoning. Stir well.
5. Pour in broth, tomatoes, beans, and pepper flakes if desired. Combine well.
6. Heat the stew to a boil then lower the heat to low.
7. Put a lid on the pot and simmer for one hour until the pork is tender to a fork's touch.
8. Ladle the stew into bowls over steaming brown rice or add the rice right into the stew.

Rainbow Fillets Almandine

Makes two servings.

Ingredients:

- 8 oz. rainbow trout, filleted
- 2 tbsp cornmeal, yellow
- 1 tbsp almonds, ground
- 1 tbsp parsley, fresh   and chopped
- 1/4 tsp celery seeds, ground
- 1/4 tsp black pepper, ground
- dash of sea salt
- 2 tsp olive, oil, Extra virgin
- 1 tbsp yogurt, nonfat
- 2 orange slices for garnish

Procedure:

1. Rinse the fillets. Check to make sure all of the bones are removed. Gently pat dry with a paper towel.
2. In a large dish, mix the cornmeal, almond meal, celery seed, and parsley.
3. Thinly coat both sides of the fillets with the yogurt.
4. Dredge fillets in meal mixture, coating both sides.
5. Heat the oil in a frying pan. When the oil is hot, gently drop fish in and cook fish for three minutes on each side. Fillets should be easy to flake with a fork and have a nice brown crisp coating.
6. Serve with a green salad.

Ginger Beef Veggie Stir Fry

Makes six servings.

Ingredients:

- 1 lb. steak, flank, cut into strips
- 2 tsp ginger, ground
- 2 cloves garlic
- 200 ml broth, beef or vegetable, fat-free
- 75 ml hoisin sauce
- 3 tbsp soy or tamari sauce
- 1 tbsp cornstarch
- 1 tsp grape-seed or canola oil
- 1/4 tsp red pepper flakes, crushed
- 1/2 bell pepper, medium, cut in strips
- 125 ml broccoli florets, chopped
- 125 ml rice, brown & instant
- 2 stalks bok choy, 1/2 inch slices
- 1 can, small water chestnuts, sliced

Procedure:

1. Stir together the steak, ginger, and garlic in a bowl.
2. Make rice according to the package directions.
3. Stir the broth, hoisin, and soy sauces with the cornstarch in a bowl until the cornstarch dissolves.
4. Heat the oil in a wok or skillet, adding red pepper flakes.
5. Add the steak to the wok and cook, constantly stirring until browned. Remove from pan and set aside.
6. Combine the broccoli, bell pepper, and carrot in the wok, cooking over medium heat for three minutes until tender yet crisp. If the mixture is too dry, add a tablespoon or two of water.

7. Mix in the bok choy and chestnuts. Cook for another two minutes, stirring continuously.
8. With the stirring spoon, make a well in the center of the vegetables and pout the broth in.
9. Cook for two minutes until the broth thickens. Stir occasionally.
10. Add in the beef and cook for another two minutes to warm up the meat.
11. Lay the stir-fry over the rice.

Tuna Surprise

Makes two servings.

Ingredients:

- 125 ml onion, chopped fine
- 2 cloves garlic, minced
- 1/4 jalapeno pepper, minced
- 1/2 bell pepper, sliced in thin strips
- 250 ml broccoli florets, chopped fine
- 1 tomato, medium,   diced
- 5 green olives, chopped fine
- 1 can tuna, small, packed in water
- 125 ml old cheddar cheese   grated
- 250 ml brown rice, cooked
- 1 tbsp grape-seed oil
- sea salt & pepper for taste

Procedure:

1. Open the tuna and drain the water.
2. Add oil to the frying pan and heat over medium-high.
3. Add the onions, garlic, jalapeno pepper, and salt. Cook and stir for two minutes
4. Stir in the bell pepper and broccoli. Cook for two minutes and keep stirring.
5. Stir in the tomato and olives. Cook for another three minutes or until broccoli is tender to the fork.
6. Flake in the tuna fish, add the rice and stir. Lower the heat to medium-low, cover, and cook for another three minutes.
7. Lower the heat to low. Stir everything once more, then sprinkle the cheese on top. Cover and allow to sit for a minute or until the

cheese is melted.

8. Serve up hot. Add a dash of black pepper now if desired.

Refried Beans with a Twist

Makes two servings

Ingredients:

- 125 ml onion, chopped small
- 1 clove garlic, large and minced
- 1/8 tsp red pepper flakes, crushed
- 1/2 tsp cinnamon, dried
- 1/2 tsp cumin, dried
- 1/4 tsp coriander, dried
- dash of oregano
- 1/2 tsp sea salt
- 1/2 stalk celery, diced
- 1 carrot, small and diced
- 1/2 bell pepper, diced
- one Roma tomato, diced
- 250 ml black beans   drained and rinsed
- 125 ml old cheddar   grated
- 1/2 avocado,   sliced into four pieces
- 2 sprigs cilantro for garnish
- Salsa for dipping
- 2 whole wheat tortillas

Procedure:

1. Heat oil in frying pan on medium heat.
2. Add first onion, garlic, and red pepper flakes, and sauté for two minutes.
3. Stir in the spices and salt. Continue to sauté for another minute.

109

4. Mix in the celery, carrot, pepper, and tomato. Continue to stir occasionally, cooking for three minutes. Option: If the mixture is a bit dry, add two tablespoons of water or broth (not beef).
5. Add in the black beans and continue to cook until the beans are moist and soft. It might be necessary to add another tablespoon of broth or water.
6. Place tortillas on two plates. Divide the rice between the two, then the bean mixture, followed by the cheese and avocado. Roll up like a burrito and place a sprig of cilantro on top.
7. Option: Salsa can be placed right in the burrito or at the side for dipping.

Italian Style Chicken Puree

Makes 1 serving.

Ingredients:

- 1/4th cup Chicken (canned)
- 1 teaspoon Italian seasoning
- 1/8 teaspoon Pepper
- 1/8 teaspoon Salt
- 1 and 1/2 tablespoons Tomato sauce

Procedure:

1. Place all the ingredients in a small size blender. Or else, you can blend all the ingredients using the back portion of one fork till you get a soft mixture.
2. Shift it into a bowl. Then microwave it for 30 seconds.
3. If you like you can add ricotta cheese or cottage cheese which is low in fat.
4. This will make it into a lasagne type of meal.
5. Note: Every serving provides approximately 4 grams of fat, 13 grams of proteins, and 3 grams of carbohydrates.

Bean Puree and Red Pepper Enchiladas

Makes 1 serving.

Ingredients:

- Half a cup of Black beans
- 1 and 1/2 tablespoons Enchilada sauce (red)
- 2 tablespoons Red pepper (jarred roasted and finely chopped)
- 1 tablespoon protein powder (unflavored)
- 2 tablespoons Chicken broth

Procedure:

1. Put black beans, red pepper and enchilada sauce in a small size sauce pan. Warm it on medium heat.
2. Put the broth.
3. You can blend the ingredients with the hand blender or shift the things into a blender.
4. Transfer the bean puree into a bowl. Let it cool for a minute and then put the protein powder. Put half more teaspoon of enchilada sauce. It is ready to be served.
5. Note: It provides 1 gram of fat, 19 grams of proteins, and 25 grams of carbohydrates.
6. Here the carbohydrate content is more than protein content because of the beans. This is not recommended. Even then, it is suitable for the pureed part and healing phase of one's diet. Other than this phase of the diet it is advisable to pair the recipe with some high protein entree. If you increase the amount of protein powder, the texture will be gritty.

Black Beans Puree with Lime

Makes 1 serving.

Ingredients:

- 1/2 tablespoon Lime juice
- 1/4th cup rinsed Black beans
- 1/2 tablespoon Jalapenos juice (from the jarred ones)
- 1/4th cup vegetable or chicken broth
- 1 tablespoon protein powder (unflavored)

Procedure:

1. Place the beans in one small pan and heat them on medium heat. Put the lime as well as the juice from the jarred jalapenos. Keep stirring while heating. Add the chicken broth.
2. Shift the mixture to one blender or use one hand blender to prepare a smooth mixture. Transfer it into a bowl.
3. Allow it to cool a bit and then mix the protein powder. Stir well. Then serve.
4. Note: It is nearly one ounce. It provides 0 grams of fat, 10 grams of proteins, and 10 grams of carbohydrates.

Tilapia - Pan Seared

Makes 1 serving.

Ingredients:

- 1/2 tablespoon Seafood seasoning
- 2 oz thawed Tilapia fillet (if you are using the frozen ones)

Procedure:

1. Heat one non-stick pan on medium heat.
2. Coat both the sides of the thawed fish with some seafood seasoning.
3. Put in the heated pan. Cook for around 7 minutes on every side or till it is cooked properly.
4. Note: It provides approximately 1 gram of fat, 10 grams proteins, and zero grams carbohydrates.

Tilapia Coated with Parmesan

Makes 4 servings.

Ingredients:

- Half a cup of grated Parmesan cheese (non-fat)
- 4 thawed Tilapia fillets (if you are using the frozen ones)
- 1/4 teaspoon dried Thyme
- 1/8 teaspoon Salt
- 1/8 teaspoon Pepper

Procedure:

1. Heat the oven to the temperature of 350F.
2. Blot the fish with one paper towel. Put grated cheese on both sides of each fillet. Then sprinkle salt, thyme, and pepper.
3. Heat one non-stick pan on medium heat. Use the pan to cook the fish in batches. Cook each side for about 1 minute. Then transfer the fillets to one small sized casserole dish.
4. Put this dish in the heated oven. Bake them till they flake easily or for about 15 minutes.
5. Note: Every serving provides approximately 5 grams of fat, 24 grams of proteins, and 3 grams of carbohydrates.

Chicken Thighs and Cream of Mushrooms

Makes 6 servings.

Ingredients:

- 1 can or 10 oz Cream of the mushroom soup (fat-free)
- 1 lb Chicken thighs

Procedure:

1. Heat the oven to a temperature of 350F.
2. Cut off the fat from the thighs as much as possible using kitchen shears. Spread it out on one baking sheet. Then season with pepper and salt.
3. Spread the cream of the mushroom soup over the chicken thighs evenly.
4. Bake it for about 20 minutes.
5. Remove from the oven and let it cool. Take tiny bites and chew slowly.
6. Note: Every serving provides approximately 2 grams of fat, 17 grams of proteins, and 5 grams of carbohydrates.

Chicken with Lemon and Rosemary

Ingredients:

- 1 tablespoon Dijon mustard
- 2 lemons (one of them should be juiced and zested, another one should be thinly sliced)
- 2 clove of Garlic (pressed or minced)
- 1 lb Chicken thighs
- 1 tablespoon of dried Rosemary or 4 sprigs of fresh rosemary

Procedure:

1. Preheat the oven to a temperature of 425F.
2. Put the lemon juice, lemon zest, garlic and mustard in one small bowl and whisk them — season with pepper and salt.
3. Toss the rosemary, sliced lemon, mustard mixture and the chicken on a baking sheet.
4. Put one layer of chicken and spread the lemons on top.
5. Roast for about 20 to 25 minutes.
6. Note: Every serving provides approximately 2 grams of carbohydrates and 31 grams of proteins.

Barbecue Salmon

Makes 4 servings.

Ingredients:

- 4 oz thawed Salmon fillets
- 4 tablespoons BBQ sauce (low sugar)
- 2 tablespoons Grill seasoning

Procedure:

1. Thaw the salmon if you are using the frozen ones. If possible, take out the salmon and keep it aside for around 20 minutes before cooking.
2. Heat one grill pan on a stovetop on high heat. Spray some cooking spray. Lower the heat to medium. Put barbecue sauce on the fillets.
3. Place the salmon on the grill. Grill for around 5 minutes in one position. Then flip it and cook for another 3 to 4 minutes. Put some more sauce on the fillets. Sprinkle a little grill seasoning while cooking.
4. Flip once again and put some more sauce. Let it cook for 1 more minute.
5. Remove it from the heat. By then the salmon should be flaky and ready for serving.
6. Note: Every serving provides 2 grams of fat, 22 grams of proteins, and 7 grams of carbohydrates.

Tilapia with Lemon Pepper

Makes 4 servings.

Ingredients:

- 4 or 6 ounce Tilapia fillets
- 1/2 teaspoon Paprika
- 1 teaspoon Garlic (granulated otherwise fresh minced)
- One and a half teaspoons of Lemon pepper
- 1 tablespoon Olive oil
- 1/4 teaspoon Salt
- Juice of 1 lime

Procedure:

1. Preheat the oven to a temperature of 400F.
2. Take a bowl and mix all dry spices. Add the olive oil. Mix and make a paste.
3. Put the tilapia on a baking sheet. Drizzle some lime juice on it.
4. Divide the paste evenly for seasoning the fillets and place one dollop on every fillet. Then spread it with your hands or use one spoon to do so.
5. Bake till the fillet flakes when you use a fork or for a time duration of 8 minutes. You can serve it along with some steamed vegetables.
6. Note: Every serving provides approximately 5 grams of fat, 21 grams of proteins, and 2 grams of carbohydrates.

Lettuce Wraps with Chicken Asian Style

Ingredients:

- 8 oz or 1 can Bamboo shoots minced (drained)
- 8 oz or 1 can Water chestnuts minced (drained)
- 3 tbsp Sherry wine (cooking)
- 2 tbsp Hoisin sauce
- 2 tsp Soy sauce (low-sodium)
- 1 tbsp Peanut butter (unsalted)
- 2 tsp Pepper sauce (for example Sriracha)
- 1 tbsp minced Garlic
- 2 packets Sugar substitute (.035 oz each, for example Splenda)
- 1 cup Onion (minced)
- 1/2 lb Chicken breast (ground)
- 1 tsp Sesame oil (toasted)
- 1 tsp Salt
- 1 tsp minced Ginger
- 8 Butter lettuce (small leaves)
- 1 chopped Green onion
- 1 small size Cucumber (cut into 1-inch strips)

Procedure:

1. Put bamboo shoots, sherry, water chestnuts, hoisin sauce, soy sauce, pepper sauce, peanut butter, a sugar substitute in one medium-sized bowl. Mix well and keep aside.
2. Spray some cooking spray on a non-stick skillet and set it on medium heat.
3. Put the onions and cook till they become soft and fragrant or for four minutes.
4. Add garlic — Cook for 1 more minute.
5. Increase the level of heat and set it at medium-high. Put the chicken, salt, and ginger.

6. Cook for 3 or 4 minutes till it is not pink any longer. Use a wooden spoon or spatula to break the chicken while cooking.
7. Add the mixture of bamboo shoots and water chestnuts — Cook for two minutes.
8. Mix the sesame oil.
9. Then remove it from heat. Divide the mixture into 8 equal parts and place on the lettuce leaves.
10. Put the cucumber slices and green onion on top and serve.

Pork Tenderloin Asian Style

Ingredients:

- 2 tbsp Worcestershire sauce
- 1/3rd cup Soy sauce (light)
- 2 tbsp Rice vinegar
- 2 tbsp Lemon juice
- 1 tbsp Ginger
- 1/3rd cup of Brown sugar
- 4 cloves Garlic
- 1 and 1/2 tsp Pepper
- 1 tbsp dry Mustard
- 2 lbs Pork tenderloin

Procedure:

1. Mix all the ingredients in a bag which can be put in a freezer.
2. Put the tenderloin in the freezer bag. Rub the pork with marinade.
3. Refrigerate it overnight. Or else, put it in the freezer and use it later.
4. Bake at a temperature of 375 degrees for thirty to forty minutes. Or else, cook on
5. low heat in a slow cooker for four to six hours.

Balsamic Roasted Chicken

Ingredients:

- 1 Chicken whole (around 4 lbs)
- 1 tsp dried Rosemary otherwise 1 tbsp fresh rosemary
- 1 tbsp Olive oil
- 1 clove Garlic
- 1/8 tsp Black pepper (freshly ground)
- 8 sprigs Rosemary (fresh)
- 1 tsp Brown sugar
- Half a cup of Balsamic vinegar

Procedure:

1. Heat the oven beforehand to a temperature of 350 degrees.
2. Mince the garlic and rosemary in one small bowl. Loosen the skin of the chicken and rub olive oil on the flesh. Then rub the mixture of the herbs. Sprinkle some black pepper. Place 2 sprigs of rosemary in the chicken's cavity and bind the chicken.
3. Put the chicken in one roasting pan. Roast for around one hour and twenty minutes. The least internal temperature till which a whole chicken must be cooked is 165 degrees. Frequently baste with the pan juices. After the chicken is browned transfer it to one serving dish.
4. Mix the brown sugar and balsamic vinegar in one small sized saucepan. Heat it till it becomes warm and the brown sugar is dissolved. But do not boil.
5. Carve and discard the chicken's skin. Put the vinegar mixture on top of the pieces. Use the rest of the rosemary sprigs for garnishing and serve.

BBQ Chicken Pizza

Ingredients:

- 1 Pizza crust 12" (thin)
- 1 cup of Tomato sauce (with no added salt)
- 8 rings of Green pepper
- 1 sliced Tomato
- 1 cup sliced Mushrooms
- 4 lbs Chicken breast (cooked, sliced into 1" thick pieces, with all fat removed)
- 1 cup shredded Mozzarella cheese (reduced-fat)
- 4 tbsp Barbecue sauce

Procedure:

1. Heat the oven beforehand to a temperature of 400 degrees.
2. Put the sauce on the crust. Place the chicken, mushrooms, and tomato on it. Sprinkle some pepper. Drizzle the barbecue sauce and put the cheese on top of the pizza.
3. Bake for around 12 or 14 minutes.
4. Cut it into small pieces and serve.

Barbecue Roasted Salmon

Ingredients:

- 2 tbsp Lemon juice (fresh)
- 1/4th cup of Pineapple juice
- 4 fillets of Salmon (6 oz each)
- 2 tbsp Brown sugar
- 2 tsp Lemon rind (grated)
- 4 tsp Chilli powder
- 1/2 tsp Salt
- 3/4 tsp ground Cumin
- 1/4 tsp Cinnamon

Procedure:

1. Heat the oven beforehand to a temperature of 400 degrees.
2. Mix the pineapple juice and lemon juice with the salmon fillets in a Ziploc bag. Put them in the fridge and marinate them for 1 hour. Turn them occasionally. Take out the salmon from the bag. Discard the marinade.
3. Mix the rest of the ingredients. Rub them over the fish. Put the fillets in a baking dish which has a coating of cooking spray.
4. Then bake them for 12 or 15 minutes. Garnish with lemon rind and serve.

Brown Rice and Black Bean Casserole

Ingredients:

- 1/3rd cup of Brown rice
- 2 cups shredded Swiss cheese (low fat)
- 1/3rd cup Onion (diced)
- 1 thinly sliced, medium sized Zucchini
- 1/4 tsp Cayenne pepper
- 1 lb cooked Chicken breast (cut in small pieces)
- Half a cup of sliced Mushrooms
- 15 oz or 1 can of drained Black beans
- 4 oz or 1 can of diced Green Chilies
- 1 cup of Vegetable Broth
- 1/2 tsp Cumin
- 1/3rd cup Carrots (shredded)
- 1 tbsp Olive oil

Procedure:

1. Combine the vegetable broth with the rice in one pot and boil. When it starts boiling, reduce the heat, cover it and simmer till the rice becomes tender or for 45 minutes.
2. Heat the oven beforehand to a temperature of 350 degrees.
3. Grease one big casserole dish lightly with some cooking spray.
4. Then heat the olive oil on medium heat in a skillet and cook the onions till they become tender.
5. Add the chicken, mushrooms, zucchini, and seasonings.
6. Stir and cook till the zucchini becomes slightly brown and the chicken is warmed up.
7. Mix the onions, cooked rice, zucchini, mushrooms, chicken, beans, carrots, chilies, and one cup of Swiss cheese in a big bowl.
8. Transfer to the casserole dish which you have prepared, and sprinkle the remaining cup of Swiss cheese.

9. Then cover the casserole with a foil and bake for thirty minutes.
10. After that, remove the cover and bake for 10 minutes.

Braised Chicken and Mushrooms

Ingredients:

- 1/4th cup of All-purpose flour (plain)
- 1/2 tsp Black pepper (freshly ground)
- 2 halves of Chicken breast (around 3/4 lb, each should be cut into half crosswise to make 4 pieces)
- 2 Chicken thighs (3/4 lb)
- 2 Chicken legs (3/4 lb)
- 1 chopped Shallot (about 1 tbsp)
- 1 lb Button mushrooms (small white)
- 1/2 lb Pearl onions (peeled)
- Half a cup of Port or Red wine (dry)
- 3/4th cup of low-sodium broth, vegetable stock or chicken stock
- 2 tbsp Balsamic vinegar
- 1/4 tsp Salt
- 2 tbsp fresh Thyme (chopped) and sprigs for garnishing
- 1 and 1/2 tbsp Canola oil or Olive oil

Procedure:

1. Mix 1/4th teaspoon of pepper with the flour in one shallow dish. Dredge the pieces of chicken in this flour.
2. Heat oil on medium to high heat in a Dutch oven or a big heavy saucepan. Put the chicken in it. Cook for 5 minutes till it becomes brown on both the sides. While cooking, turn it once. After that, transfer it to one platter.
3. Put the shallot in the pan. Sauté for a minute till it becomes soft. Then add and saute the mushrooms for 3 or 4 minutes till they become slightly brown. Next, add and saute the onions for 2 or 3 minutes till they become brownish.
4. Pour the wine and stock in the pan and deglaze it. Stir with one wooden spoon and scrape the browned bits. Put the pieces of

chicken in it and boil. When it starts boiling cover it and decrease the heat. Let it simmer for 45 or 50 minutes till the vegetables and chicken become tender. Add the vinegar, one teaspoon salt, 1/4th teaspoon pepper, and chopped thyme.

5. To serve put the vegetables in separate shallow bowls. Place 2 chicken pieces on top of each of the servings. Use thyme sprigs to garnish them.

Broccoli Baked with Cheddar

Ingredients:

- Half a cup of Onions (chopped finely)
- 4 cups fresh Broccoli (chopped)
- One and a half cup of Egg substitute
- 2 tbsp Water
- 1/2 tsp Black pepper (ground)
- 1 cup Cheddar cheese (shredded)
- 1 cup Milk (fat-free)

Procedure:

1. Heat the oven beforehand to a temperature of 350 degrees. Coat one baking dish lightly with some cooking spray.
2. Combine the onions, broccoli, and water in one non-stick skillet. Sauté them on medium heat for 5 or 8 minutes till they become tender. Add water if needed but try to use the least amount of water. When they are cooked, drain the water and keep them aside.
3. Mix 3/4th cup of cheese, milk, and egg substitute in one bowl. Add pepper and broccoli mixture. Stir well.
4. Put the mixture in the baking dish you have prepared. Place the dish in a big pan which is filled with around 1" of water.
5. Bake without covering the dish for 45 minutes.
6. Then take it out of the oven. Put the rest of the cheese on top of it. Allow it to stand for 10 minutes and then serve.

Broccoli Baked with Cheese and Egg

Ingredients:

- 6 big Eggs
- 4 oz light Margarine
- 6 tbsp Flour
- 1/2 lb Cheddar cheese (low-fat)
- 1 pinch Black pepper
- 2 lbs Cottage cheese (non-fat)
- 10 oz frozen Broccoli (thawed and chopped)
- 1 tsp Salt
- 1 pinch Paprika (optional)
- Half a cup of sliced Mushrooms, canned or fresh (optional)
- 4 oz chopped Pimento (optional)

Procedure:

1. Heat the oven beforehand to a temperature of 350 degrees.
2. Mix all the ingredients.
3. Spray a casserole dish (2-quart) with some cooking spray.
4. Put the mixture of ingredients in the pan you have prepared. Bake for ninety minutes. Serve when it is hot.

Broiled Grouper and Teriyaki Sauce

Ingredients:

- 1 tbsp Teriyaki sauce (reduced-sodium)
- 2 (4 oz each) Grouper fillets
- 2 wedges of Lemon
- 1/2 tsp minced Garlic
- 1/4 tsp Italian seasoning

Procedure:

1. Put the garlic and teriyaki sauce in one small bowl and whisk them.
2. Spray one baking pan lightly with some cooking spray. Put the fillets in it. Brush the sides of grouper fillets with teriyaki marinade. Cover and keep them in the fridge for a minimum of 15 minutes to marinate.
3. Heat the broiler or grill beforehand. Place the rack at a distance of 4" from the source of heat.
4. Broil or grill for about 5 or 10 minutes. After that, remove the fillets from the grill. Squeeze one lemon wedge on each fillet. Sprinkle the Italian seasoning and serve.

Stuffed Chicken with Spinach, Pepper Cheese and Cajun

Ingredients:

- 1 lb Chicken breasts
- 1 cup Spinach frozen and thawed (or else fresh cooked)
- 1 tbsp Bread crumbs
- 3 oz shredded Pepper cheese (reduced-fat)
- 2 tbsp Cajun seasoning
- Toothpicks

Procedure:

1. Heat the oven beforehand to a temperature of 350 degrees.
2. Make the chicken flat so that it is 1/4" thick.
3. Combine pepper cheese, salt, and spinach in one medium-sized bowl.
4. Mix the bread crumbs and Cajun seasoning in one small bowl.
5. Put about 1/4th cup of spinach mixture on every chicken breast with a spoon. Roll each one tightly. Fasten them with several toothpicks.
6. Brush all of them with olive oil. Then sprinkle Cajun seasoning over all of them.
7. Sprinkle the remaining cheese and spinach on top (optional).
8. Keep the seam-side of the chicken up on a baking sheet lined with one tin foil so that it is easy to clean later.
9. Bake for 35 - 40 minutes.
10. Make sure that you take out all the toothpicks before serving. Slice them into medallions or serve whole.

Acorn Squash Cheesy and Stuffed

Ingredients:

- 1 lb extra-lean Turkey breast (ground)
- 2 seeded and halved Acorn squash
- 1 cup Celery (diced)
- 1 cup Onion (finely chopped)
- 1 cup sliced Mushrooms (fresh)
- 1 tsp Basil
- 1 tsp Oregano
- 1 pinch Black pepper (ground)
- 1/8 tsp Salt
- 8 oz Tomato sauce (1 can)
- 1 cup Cheddar cheese (shredded)
- 1 tsp Garlic powder

Procedure:

1. Heat the oven beforehand to a temperature of 350 degrees.
2. Put the squash in one glass dish in such a way that the cut side is down.
3. Cook on high for twenty minutes in the microwave till it becomes almost tender.
4. Brown the ground turkey in one non-stick pan on medium heat.
5. Add onions and celery and sauté them.
6. Put the mushrooms and cook for another 2 or 3 minutes.
7. Add the dry seasonings and tomato sauce.
8. Divide the mixture into 4 portions. Put it in the squash with a spoon and cover.
9. Cook for fifteen minutes in an oven which has already been heated to 350 degrees.
10. After that, remove the cover and sprinkle the cheese. Then once again keep it in
11. oven till the cheese starts bubbling.

Vegetarian Cheesy Chilli

Ingredients:

- 2 cloves of Garlic
- 1 diced large Bell pepper (green)
- 1 cup chopped Onions
- 1/2 lb sliced Mushrooms
- 8 oz Tomato sauce
- 1 can or 14.5 oz diced Tomatoes otherwise 2 cups of fresh tomatoes
- 2 tsp Olive oil
- 1 medium-sized thinly sliced Zucchini
- 2 tbsp Chilli powder
- 2 cans or 15 oz rinsed Kidney beans (red)
- 1 cup Cheddar cheese (shredded)
- 1 packet or 10 oz frozen Corn

Procedure:

1. Heat garlic and olive oil in a big pan.
2. Add mushroom, onions, and green pepper. Cook till they become tender.
3. Put the tomato sauce, chili powder, and diced tomatoes and boil.
4. When it starts boiling turn down the heat to low and add the kidney beans and
5. zucchini. Simmer for ten to fifteen minutes.
6. Add the corn and half a cup of cheddar cheese and stir.
7. Simmer for another ten to fifteen minutes.
8. After it is cooked put the remaining cheddar cheese on top and serve.

Chicken Casserole

Ingredients:

- 1 cup Chicken breast (cubed and cooked)
- 2 cups Mixed vegetables (frozen)
- Half a cup of uncooked Wheat pasta otherwise 1 cup of cooked wheat pasta
- 1 can or 10.5 oz cream of the Chicken soup (98% free of fat)
- 1 cup reduced-fat Cheddar cheese (shredded)
- 3/4th cup of water
- 4 oz canned Mushrooms
- Pepper, onion powder and garlic powder according to taste

Procedure:

1. Heat the oven beforehand to a temperature of 350 degrees.
2. Spray one casserole dish (9x3) with some cooking spray.
3. Then cook the vegetables and pasta according to the directions given on the
4. packages.
5. Combine the chicken, mushrooms, half a cup of cheese, soup, cooked vegetables
6. and pasta and water in a big bowl.
7. Add pepper, onion powder and garlic powder according to taste.
8. Put this mixture into the casserole dish which has been greased. Sprinkle the
9. remaining cheese on it.
10. Bake it for 25 or 30 minutes till the cheese becomes bubbly and golden brown.

Chicken Cheese Wrap

Ingredients:

- One whole wheat Tortilla (low-carb)
- 1/4 lb Chicken breast (all visible fat removed)
- 1/4th cup of chopped Onions
- 1/4th cup of sliced Green pepper
- 1/4th cup of sliced Mushrooms
- 1 wedge or 3/4 lb Swiss cheese (light)
- 2 tsp sliced pickled spicy Chilli peppers (according to taste)

Procedure:

1. Flatten the chicken breast and make it 4-inch thick. Cut it into thin strips.
2. Place a pan on medium to high heat. Mist it with some cooking spray.
3. Put the onions and chicken in it and cook till the onions become translucent and
4. the chicken is not pink anymore.
5. Add the mushrooms and green peppers and cook till they become soft.
6. Place the tortilla in between 2 moist paper towels and microwave for twenty seconds.
7. Put one strip of cheese in the center of the tortilla when it is warm.
8. Then put chicken, mushrooms, peppers, and onions on top of it.
9. If you are using chili peppers, then put them also.
10. Fold the sides of the tortilla over the middle part and then serve.

Chicken Fajitas

Ingredients:

- 1/4th cup of Lime juice
- 3 lb Chicken breasts (1/4" strips)
- 1-2 cloves of Garlic (minced)
- 1/2 slivered Green bell pepper (sweet)
- 1 tsp Chilli powder
- 1/2 slivered Red bell pepper (sweet)
- 1/2 tsp Cumin (ground)
- 1 big sliced onion
- 12 Tortillas 8" each (whole wheat)
- Half a cup of Salsa
- Half a cup of Sour cream (fat-free)
- Half a cup of Shredded Cheese

Procedure:

1. Combine the lime juice, garlic, chili powder, and cumin in one big bowl. Add the
2. chicken slices. Stir till they are well coated.
3. Then marinate them for fifteen minutes.
4. Cook the chicken in a pan on the stovetop or grill for three minutes.
5. Put the peppers and onions and cook for 3 or 5 minutes.
6. Divide the mixture equally among all the tortillas.
7. Put two teaspoons of salsa, two teaspoons of shredded cheese and two teaspoons
8. of sour cream on top of each one. Roll them up and then serve.

Chicken Rollatini and Spinach with Parmesan

Ingredients:

- 8 cutlets of Chicken breast (3 oz each)
- 6 tbsp egg whites
- Half a cup of whole wheat seasoned Bread crumbs (Italian seasoning)
- 1/4th cup Parmesan cheese (grated)
- 5 oz frozen and thawed Spinach (squeezed dry)
- 6 tbsp Ricotta cheese (part skim)
- 6 oz shredded Mozzarella (part skim)
- 1 cup of Marinara sauce
- Non-stick cooking spray

Procedure:

1. Heat the oven beforehand to a temperature of 450 degrees.
2. Spray a baking dish (9x13) made of glass with non-stick cooking spray.
3. Use pepper and salt to season the chicken cutlets.
4. Mix 2 tablespoons of parmesan cheese with the bread crumbs in one small bowl.
5. In another bowl put 4 tablespoons of egg whites.
6. Combine the ricotta cheese, 1.5 oz mozzarella, spinach, remaining parmesan cheese and 2 remaining tablespoons of egg whites.
7. Put 2 tablespoons of this mixture on every seasoned cutlet.
8. Roll all the cutlets loosely. Use 1 or 2 toothpicks to secure each of them.
9. Dip these rolls in the egg whites and then in the mixture of bread crumbs. Place them in the baking dish which has been greased. Keep them in such a way that the seam side is down.
10. Spray the chicken rollatini's light with non-stick spray.
11. Bake for 25 minutes.

12. Take it out of the oven and put the remaining mozzarella cheese, and marinara sauce on top.
13. Bake for another 3 minutes till the cheese melts and starts bubbling.
14. Serve with parmesan cheese and some more sauce on the side.

Stir Fry Chicken with Basil and Eggplant

Ingredients:

- 1/4th cup of fresh Basil (coarsely chopped)
- 2 tbsp fresh mint (chopped)
- 3/4th cup of Broth or Chicken stock (low-sodium)
- 3 spring or Green Onions, 2 chopped coarsely and 1 sliced thinly
- 2 cloves of Garlic
- 1 tbsp fresh Ginger (chopped)
- 2 tbsp Olive oil (extra-virgin)
- 1 Eggplant (small)
- 1 coarsely chopped yellow Onion
- 1 Bell pepper (red)
- 1 Bell pepper (yellow)
- 1 lb Chicken breasts (2" long and 1/2" wide strips)
- 2 tbsp Soy sauce (low-sodium)

Procedure:

1. Put mint, basil, ginger, one-fourth cup of stock, green onions (chopped) and garlic in a food processor or blender. Blend and mince the mixture but do not make it into a puree. Keep it aside.
2. Heat one tablespoon of olive oil in one big non-stick pan on medium to high heat. Put the eggplant, bell peppers and yellow onion and saute for 8 minutes till they become tender. Transfer them into a bowl. Cover them with one kitchen towel.
3. Put 1 tablespoon of olive oil in the pan. Heat it over medium to high heat. Saute the mixture you made earlier, in it for 1 minute. Stir constantly. Then put chicken strips and soy sauce. Saute them for 2 minutes. Put half a cup of stock in the pan. Cook till it starts boiling. Add eggplant mixture and cook for 3 minutes. Then transfer it to one serving dish. Garnish with green onion and serve.

Chili

Ingredients:

- 1 lb extra-lean Beef (ground)
- Half a cup of chopped Onions
- 2 big Tomatoes otherwise 2 cups of unsalted canned tomatoes
- 1 cup Celery (chopped)
- 4 cups of rinsed Kidney beans (canned)
- 1 and 1/2 tbsp Chilli powder
- 1 tsp Sugar
- 2 tbsp Cornmeal
- Water as much as needed
- Jalapeno peppers (optional)

Procedure:

1. Put the onions and ground beef in one soup pot. Sauté on medium heat till the onion becomes translucent and the beef becomes brown.
2. Add the kidney beans, tomatoes, celery, chili powder, and sugar to the meat mixture and cover it. Cook for ten minutes and stir frequently. Remove the cover and put as much water as needed. Put the cornmeal. Then cook for a minimum of 10 more minutes and let the flavors blend.
3. Take out into serving bowls. Use jalapeno peppers for garnishing.

Cod with Capers and Lemon

Ingredients:

- 4 (6 oz each) Cod fillets
- 1 tsp low-sodium Bouillon granules (chicken-flavored)
- 1 cup of hot Water
- 1 tbsp soft Butter
- 2 Lemons
- 4 tsp rinsed Capers
- 1 tbsp plain all-purpose Flour

Procedure:

1. Heat the oven beforehand to a temperature of 350 degrees.
2. Spray 4 foil squares with some cooking spray.
3. Put 1 fillet on every foil square. Cut a lemon into half. Squeeze out the juice of one
4. half on the fish and cut the second half into slices. Put these on the fillets and close
5. the foils
6. Place them in the oven. Bake for 20 minutes.
7. Take out the peel of the other lemon and cut it into quarter inch wide strips.
8. In one small bowl mix the hot water and the bouillon granules. Stir till they dissolve.
9. Mix the flour and butter in another bowl. Transfer them to one heavy saucepan. Place it over medium heat and stir until the mixture melts. Put the bouillon and keep stirring till it thickens. Then put the capers. Remove from heat. Serve on the fillets. Use the lemon peel to garnish them.

Chicken with Greek Yogurt

Ingredients:

- 4 (4 oz each) Chicken breasts
- 1 tsp Garlic powder
- 1 cup Greek yogurt (plain)
- Half a cup of Parmesan cheese (grated)
- 1/2 tsp Pepper
- One and a half teaspoons of seasoning

Procedure:

1. Heat the oven beforehand to a temperature of 375 degrees.
2. Mix Greek yogurt, seasonings, and cheese in a bowl.
3. Put a lining of foil in a baking sheet and spray some cooking spray.
4. Coat the yogurt mixture on all the chicken breasts. Then place them on the foil in the baking sheet.
5. Bake for 45 minutes.

Magic Moist Chicken

Ingredients:

- 3 lb Chicken breasts
- One and a quarter cups of whole wheat bread crumbs (Italian)
- Half a cup of light Mayonnaise

Procedure:

1. Heat the oven beforehand to a temperature of 425 degrees.
2. Brush the mayonnaise on the chicken.
3. Put the bread crumbs in a big plate. Roll the chicken in the crumbs till it gets coated.
4. Then place the chicken on the foil in the pan. Bake for forty to 45 minutes.

Chicken with Taco Filling

Ingredients:

- 1 lb Chicken breasts
- One cup of Chicken broth
- One packet containing 1.25 oz Taco seasoning

Procedure:

1. Mix the taco seasoning and the chicken broth in one bowl.
2. Place the chicken in a slow cooker.
3. Put the seasoning mixture and the broth on the chicken.
4. Cover it and cook for 6 or 8 hours on low heat.
5. Shred the chicken.
6. Cook for another 30 minutes so that the excess juices are absorbed.
7. Serve as a topping for some salad, filling for the tacos, or on its own as a source of protein.

Snacks

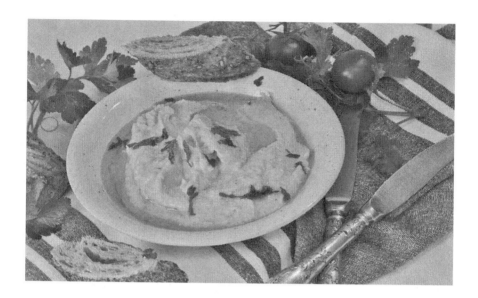

Hummus

Ingredients:

- 1 can chickpeas, drained and rinsed
- 1 tbsp peanut butter
- 1/2 lemon, juice only
- 1 tsp lemon rind, minced
- 1 tsp salt
- 1/4 tsp red pepper flakes, crushed
- 1 tbsp olive oil
- 1 clove garlic
- Option, substitute pesto for peanut butter

Procedure:

1. Place everything in the food processor. Start to puree while slowly drizzling in two tablespoons of water. Puree until exceptionally creamy.
2. Place in a bowl and keep cool in the fridge until ready to enjoy with any chopped, sliced, or whole vegetable of your choice. These could include sweet bell peppers, cherry tomatoes, radishes, fennel, jicama, and snap peas.

Cheese Chips

Sure to satisfy any chip craving with this three-ingredient mix.

Ingredients:

- 10 tbsp parmesan cheese shredded
- garlic powder
- 2 tbsp fresh basil finely chopped

Procedure:

1. Heat the oven to 350 degrees. Line a baking sheet with parchment paper.
2. Scoop one tablespoon of cheese and drop in a plop on the baking sheet.
3. With your fingers, gently spread the cheese into a thin circle and add a pinch of garlic powder and a pinch of basil.
4. Repeat until all of the cheese is gone.
5. Place sheet in oven until circle edges are golden brown. Give them a minute to cool.

Desserts

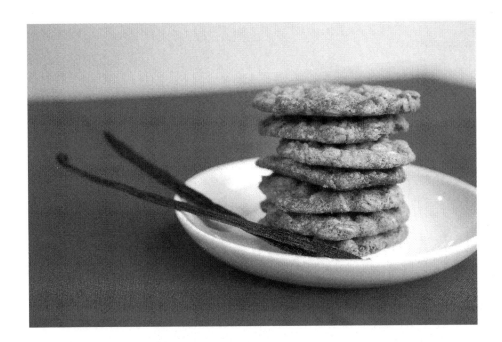

Peanut Butter Joy Cookies

Makes eighteen cookies.

Ingredients:

- 250 ml quick oats
- 250 ml peanut butter, unsweetened
- 250 ml Splenda
- 1 tsp vanilla
- 1/2 tsp cinnamon, dried
- 1 egg

Procedure:

- Pre-heat oven to 350 degrees.
- Place the peanut butter and Splenda in a mixing bowl. Using a sturdy spoon or hand beaters, beat the two together until smooth.
- Add in the egg, keep mixing, then add the vanilla.
- Last, add in the oats and cinnamon. Continue to mix until everything is nice smooth dough.
- Scoop the dough out a by dessert spoon and using your hands, roll into balls. Place the balls on a cookie sheet and squish them gently down with a fork.
- Place cookies in the oven for eight minutes until golden brown. Wait for them to cool before lifting off the pan.

Chocolate Almond Ginger Mousse

Makes five servings.

Ingredients:

- 325 ml milk, skim & cold
- 1 instant pudding package (for four servings), fat-free and sugar-free
- 250 ml Cool Whip Lite, thawed out
- 1/4 tsp ginger, dried
- 1 tbsp almonds, sliced

Procedure:

1. Pour cold milk into a mixing bowl.
2. Beating steadily with wire whisk, add the pudding mix and dried ginger. Keep whisking for two minutes.
3. Fold in the Cool Whip topping.
4. Spoon into five pudding cups, refrigerate until needed. Garnish with sliced almonds just before serving.

Bella's Apple Crisp

Makes 4 servings.

Ingredients:

- Four apples, hard and crisp, cored and sliced
- 1/2 lemon
- 2 tbsp water
- 2 tbsp agave nectar or one tbsp honey

Ingredients for Toppings:
- 200 ml old-fashioned rolled oats
- 2 tbsp butter, cold
- 1/2 tsp cinnamon
- 125 ml chopped walnuts

Procedure:

1. Heat oven to 350 degrees.
2. Place sliced apples in the bottom of an eight-inch pie plate or square cake pan.
3. Drizzle the water, lemon juice, and syrup over the apples.
4. In a mixing bowl, stir together the oats and cinnamon. Use a pastry cutter or two knives to cut in the butter mixture until it resembles coarse breadcrumbs.
5. Stir in the chopped nuts.
6. Sprinkle the mixture over the apples covering them completely.
7. Cover pan with tin foil and slide into the middle of the oven for twenty minutes.
8. Remove tin foil from pan and continue to bake for another ten to fifteen minutes until topping is golden brown.
9. Option: Serve with a dab of fat-free, sugar-free ice cream.

Red Energy Wonders

Makes around sixteen ball-shaped treats.

Ingredients:

- 325 ml coconut, shredded and divided into a 225 ml portion and a 100 ml portion
- 125 ml oats, rolled
- 125 ml of strawberries
- 125 ml almonds
- 4 dates, Medjool, pit-less
- 75 ml almond butter

Procedure:

1. Place the 225 portions of coconut and all the rest of the ingredients in a food processor. On high speed, process until smooth and fully mixed.
2. Pour the remaining coconut onto a plate. With a spoon, scoop out one tablespoon of the mixture and form into a ball. Roll this ball around in the coconut, then place on a plate lined with parchment paper. Repeat until all of the mixtures are used.
3. Place the plate in the fridge for at least two hours before serving. Keep Energy Wonders in an airtight container in the fridge.

Apple Rhubarb Popsicle Treats

Makes 4 treats

Ingredients:

- 500 ml rhubarb, diced
- 1 snack cup applesauce, unsweetened
- 2 tsp agave syrup or sugar

Procedure:

1. Place the rhubarb slices in a little water over medium heat on your stove. Cover and cook while occasionally stirring until it becomes a mush.
2. Remove from heat and stir in the applesauce and syrup.
3. Ladle into Popsicle forms or small snack size zip lock bags. Place in the freezer to set.

Greek Yogurt and Strawberry Whip

Makes 6 servings.

Ingredients:

- 3 Strawberries (frozen)
- 2/3rd Plain Greek yogurt (zero percent fat)
- 1 tablespoon Natural sweetener (no calorie)
- Half a cup of lightly whipped topping

Procedure:

1. Place the strawberries in some small bowl which can be used in the microwave. Defrost them for about 60 seconds.
2. Use the kitchen shears to dice them till they are chopped nicely and become slightly runny. Add the Greek yogurt. Stir well.
3. Add the sweetener after that and stir once again. Add the lightly whipped topping.
4. You can serve it immediately or else cover it and keep in the fridge. It may be eaten as a dip or alone.
5. Note: Every serving provides approximately 1 gram of fat, 2 grams of proteins, and 3 grams of carbohydrates.

Chocolate and Protein Pudding

Makes 4 servings.

Ingredients:

- 2 tablespoons Chocolate protein powder (whey)
- 1 cup Greek yogurt (zero percent fat)

Procedure:

1. Put all the ingredients in a bowl and use a rubber spatula to mix them. Stir till they are well blended.
2. Note: Every serving provides approximately zero grams of fat, 13 grams of proteins, and 4 grams of carbohydrates.

Creamy Sugar-Free Gelatin Squares

Ingredients:

- 1 packet or 0.6-ounce Gelatin (sugar-free, whichever flavor you like)
- 1 and 1/2 cup boiling water
- 1 cup of cold water
- Ice cubes as much as needed
- 1 and 1/2 cup Whipped topping (light and thawed)

Procedure:

1. Mix the gelatin with the boiling water in a big bowl. Stir till it is completely dissolved.
2. Put enough ice in the cold water and make 1 and 1/2 cup of water.
3. Add this ice water to the gelatin. Keep stirring till the ice melts completely.
4. Take out 1 and 1/2 cup of gelatin and put it on the counter. Keep the remaining gelatin in the fridge till it becomes slightly thick or for 30 minutes.
5. Put ¾ of a cup of whipped topping on the thickened gelatin. Then whisk till it is well blended.
6. Then pour it into an 8" square shaped dish. Put it in the fridge for 30 minutes or till the gelatin sets but does not become firm.
7. After that pour the reserved gelatin on the creamy layer of gelatin in the dish.
8. Refrigerate till it becomes firm or for 3 hours. Then cut it into squares and put the rest of the whipped topping on it.

Ricotta and Sugar-Free Strawberry Gelatin

Makes 4 servings

Ingredients:

- 1 packet Strawberry gelatin (sugar-free, any flavor can be used)
- 1 cup of boiling water
- 2/3rd cup Ricotta cheese (light)
- 1 cup of cold water

Procedure:

1. Use one fork for fluffing up the cheese. Prepare 4 dishes for pouring the mixture.
2. Pour the contents of the gelatin packet in a medium-sized mixing bowl. Put 1 cup of boiling water and whisk till the gelatin dissolves completely. Mix the ricotta cheese.
3. Put cold water. Mix all the things. Pour the mixture into the dishes you have prepared. Cover them and refrigerate till it sets or for at least 2 hours.
4. Remove and throw away the topmost layer of gelatin till the darker colored, and dense gelatin becomes visible.
5. Note: Every serving provides approximately 2 grams of fat, 5 grams of proteins, and 1 gram of carbohydrates.

Peaches and Cottage Cheese

Ingredients:

- Fresh peaches (sliced)
- Cottage cheese

Procedure:

1. Remove the skin of the peaches and slice them.
2. Put some cottage cheese on the peaches and serve. Enjoy the taste of cheese and fruit in each bite.

Apple Squash Bake

Ingredients:

- 1 Butternut Squash (medium size, peeled, cut as 3/4" cubes)
- 2 Apples (medium size, peeled and cored, cut as thin wedges)
- 2 tsp Cinnamon (ground)
- 1 tbsp Splenda
- 1/4th cup Butter (melted)
- 1/3rd tsp Salt
- 1 tbsp all-purpose Flour

Procedure:

1. Mix the apples and squash in one casserole dish.
2. Combine the rest of the ingredients and put over the apples and squash. Then mix everything.
3. Cover it and bake for fifty to sixty minutes at a temperature of 350 degrees.
4. If you want the topping to be crispier, remove the lid of the dish for 10 minutes when cooking is coming to an end.

Pumpkin Mousse

Ingredients:

- 1 can or 15 oz Pumpkin
- 1 packet or 4 oz Vanilla pudding (fat-free)
- 2 cups of whipped Topping (sugar-free)
- Half a cup of Skim Milk
- 1 tsp Cinnamon
- Allspice, clove, ginger, Splenda, and nutmeg, to taste

Procedure:

1. Mix all the ingredients.
2. Whip till they become creamy and smooth.
3. Note: One cup of this recipe provides approximately 4.4 grams of fat, 2 grams of protein, and 28 grams of carbohydrates.

Tasty Cottage Cheese Treat

Ingredients:

- 2 containers of 24 oz Cottage cheese (fat-free)
- 1 container of 8 oz Whipped Topping (sugar-free)
- 2 packages of 3 oz Gelatin (sugar-free, flavor according to choice)

Procedure:

1. Mix all the ingredients in one big bowl.
2. Add some fruit of your choice. (optional)
3. Note: One cup of this recipe provides approximately 3 grams of fat, 22 grams of proteins, and 24 grams of carbohydrates.

Chapter 6: Maximizing Your Post-Surgery Life

While deciding to have the surgery, making it through the initial recovery period is certainly not going to be a walk in the park. The real journey begins once you come out the other side and can approach life in a more-or-less healthy fashion. What follows is a variety of tips and tricks handpicked to help ensure that the next phase of your life is the best phase of your life. One of these blocks which are essential to your ongoing quality of life is a positive recognition of your choice and the daily achievements you will be making. You are following a nutrient-rich diet without including a lot of empty calories. You are enjoying more activity in your day and perhaps have a new friend or two as a result. Now, it is time to celebrate your new life.

The new you: First things first, stop, take a breath, and enjoy your new physique. You have likely been so busy following all the rules and walking on eggshells while everything was healing, it is entirely possible you have made it this far without even celebrating how good you now look. However, while it is true that weight loss comes with an overwhelming sense of achievement, it is vital that before you rush out and buy a brand-new wardrobe, you pause and consider a few things.

First, you will have a new physical reality of leftover skin, the largest organ in the human body, which was stretched before your new life path. This extra skin can be a source of discomfort, rashes, and even pain. It is a normal by-product of the Gastric Sleeve surgery. The loose skin means that you are losing weight in all of the places you should be. By maintaining the healthy lifestyle choices, you have set out for yourself and proper care, the skin will revert to its original tautness.

You may find the excess skin unsightly. You should learn and acknowledge that your body takes more time to heal and stabilize than it takes a computer to log onto Netflix. There are a few options you have to encourage the healing process. Additionally, these options feel luxurious all on their own and are a good way to celebrate and pamper the new you.

Massages will tighten the skin as they encourage an increase in the circulation of your blood and lymph tissues. The increased circulation assists your body in the removal of cellular by-products, encourages a taut skin surface, stimulates your ability for relaxation through lowering your blood pressure, thus creating a calmer and more patient you. It is a lovely reward for all of the hard work you are engaged in.

A scrub with sea salts is known to increase your blood flow, and over time, it will tighten your skin. Showering twice a day using a high-quality sea salt scrub throughout a couple of weeks is the best way to achieve this.

Conversely, swimming in a chlorinated pool is not recommended as the chemical chlorine will dry your skin out and can damage the skin cells themselves. If you can locate a saltwater pool, this would be the more beneficial option to choose. Make sure you shower well after swimming and use a natural moisturizer containing vitamins and collagen.

Beware that if over time, you are still maintaining a significant amount of loose skin, you might want to consult with your doctor about the use of body contouring. This is where you access the services of a plastic surgeon who will surgically remove excess skin, re-attaching it following the contours of your body. Given the financial cost and health risks associated with multiple surgeries, I would recommend trying the tips above with a generous dose of time and patience before taking this route.

Once you feel you are on the right path with your the re-shaping of your skin, purchasing new clothes will be essential and rewarding. I advise you not to get overly excited and buy a whole wardrobe in the first three months. Avoid purchasing dream clothes or one-day-I-will-fit-into-this outfits. Buying a few choice items at a time allows you to balance out what is happening with the changes in your body with the changes in your wardrobe. Given the time involved in developing a new lifestyle, you might surprise yourself with what you end up doing. For example, you might develop a passion for cycling, and proper bike attire will be required. Try not to make a purchase based on your old lifestyle, instead look for clothes that excite you about wearing them. They feel good, look good, and can help you move forward in recognizing who you are.

Along with the clothes, you might also want to consider changing your hairstyle. Again, be patient. Your face will be the first to show signs of weight loss but try not to rush into too drastically changing in your look. This could prove to be overwhelming as you want to recognize who you are in the mirror and adjust gradually to your changing physique. Talk to your stylist about a long-term approach to your 'look' and work together to create the image you are feeling on the inside.

Lastly, it will be of utmost importance to find a superior salesperson to assist you in the purchase of new shoes. You have probably developed a gait over the years, which reflected your body's need to support your weight. With the weight gone, you will need proper footwear to ensure you are striding forward with the best alignment you can achieve from the ground up.

Mental health: While the thought of "changing your look too quickly" might sound ridiculous at first, the fact of the matter is that you have undergone a very serious procedure in order to enact a significant lifestyle change and there very well might come a time when you don't recognize the person looking back at you. Now, this doesn't necessarily have to be a serious issue, and for some people, it will be no different that the shock of looking in the mirror the first few times after a dramatic haircut. For other's however, it has the potential to cause issues as they cannot reconcile how they feel with how they look.

Outside of personal struggles, this also has the potential to cause issues with your relationships as the experience is likely going to change you as a person and not everyone in your life is going to align with who you are when you come out the other side. While this will likely only cause your strong relationships to grow even stronger still, it can cause weak relationships to fracture and suffer as a result. Likewise, your relationships with friends and loved ones might change as the dynamics shift, and some people support you while others don't.

Again, this is not to say that everyone is going to deal with these types of issues, but as they are a possibility it is important to have access to a mental healthcare professional and check in with them from time to time for the first six months or so, just to make sure there aren't any issues that could limit your full potential moving forward.

Be prepared for rough patches: Regardless of how well things seem to be going out of the gate, however, it is also important that you mentally prepare yourself for the likelihood that you will eventually experience bumps in the road. These may be mental issues you have to sort out, relationship issues caused by yourself or others, physical issues with the recovery process or even weight loss issues caused by hitting an unexpected plateau. The specifics of the issues that affect you don't matter; what matters is that you are aware that they are coming and prepare yourself accordingly.

When it comes to physical issues, it is important to keep an open dialog with your Doctor and don't hesitate to contact them the second you feel as though something is wrong. When it comes to mental issues, you need to have a mental healthcare professional you can speak with freely and understand that issues related to personal appearance are extremely complicated and there is nothing wrong with having a hard time adjusting to a major change, especially one that happened so rapidly.

When it comes to weight loss, it is important to keep in mind that it is perfectly natural for your body to have to work harder to achieve similar results the closer you get to your ideal weight. Likewise, everyone is going to hit weight loss plateaus from time to time, and your body is more primed to them because of your previous experiences. Your body may well still be operating under the assumption that your standard weight is the weight you used to have, not the weight you are aiming for. If this is the case, then you will need to work extra hard to help it create a new ideal weight. Breaking through these preset points is what causes a plateau, and the only way to get past it is to stay the course and power through.

If you hit one of these plateaus, it is essential not to get discouraged and try to change up your diet or workout routine to spark a change. What you need to understand about the body is that it is always trying to find homeostasis. The body is endlessly trying to find a permanent home. It does not like change, so when you notice yourself hitting a plateau, you must change up what you are currently doing. Whether that may be a change up in your workout regime, changing up some of the food, you are eating, or even investing a diet plan from a professional so you know exactly how much calories you are consuming and guarantee success. Finally, don't forget that once your body has adjusted to your new stomach, one pound of weight loss per week is considered healthy so don't fret once your weight loss evens out at that amount, as it only means you are well on your way to hitting your desired weight.

Exercise

Your doctor may provide you with an exercise plan, or you may choose to consult with a personal trainer who has experience with patients with Gastric Sleeve surgery. Generally speaking, you can expect to begin with a moderate expectation, say ten minutes daily, increasing gradually over time. Once you feel confident that you are ready, you can look at several options available to you for increasing your strength, range of motion, and aerobic capability.

It is important to keep in mind that while you will certainly start to see results from simply not feeling as hungry in general and eating less overall, exercise will still play a crucial part in getting you to where you need to be. After all, diet can only take you so far when it comes to reaching your desired BMI, weight, or body fat percentage. Exercise will also help to accelerate many of the other benefits associated with the surgery, including improving your cardiovascular health and reducing your blood pressure.

Getting started: First things first, it is important to never jump into any type of exercise immediately after your surgery has been performed. While it can be easy to get frustrated, the simple fact is that healing takes time, and if you push too hard too fast, you will only end up doing more harm than good. Likewise, you will want to take great care to avoid adding any new exercise to your plan without consulting your Doctor first.

Within the first month after having the surgery, it is common for many people to feel quite uncomfortable. During this time many surgeons recommend a simple walking program where patients are recommended to walk for 5 - 10 minutes, three times per day

Other types of exercise should be avoided during this time with resistance training exercises being especially constrained.

2-3 months

The amount of exercise that can be undertaken during this period is often going to depend on your overall fitness before the surgery. Regardless, it is likely that sometime before 90 days you will be cleared for slightly more strenuous activities, with water-based exercises proving quite popular on average. Many people find this a great choice as it puts limited stress on the joins and many movements are easier to perform in the water. All activity level during this period should never become so intense that a conversation cannot be easily maintained at the same time.

4 months and beyond

By this point, you will be able to engage in a wide variety of normal activities which means that, with your Doctor's permission, you can start working more on building your core strength and overall wellness.

Finally, it is also important to be cautious when it comes to activities that require significant coordination and balance because the surgery has likely led to a change in your center of balance which can make these exercises more difficult or potentially dangerous than they otherwise would be.

Setting the right goals

Setting the right goals for yourself post-surgery is an important step in ensuring that all of your hard work and sacrifice up to this point doesn't end up being all for anything. Unfortunately, as you likely spent quite some time with the idea of gastric sleeve surgery as your end goal, it can be hard to readjust your priorities and ensure everything keeps moving forward as it should. One way to help you ensure that the goals you set moving forward are as relevant as they are motivating, is to double check that they are **SMART** as well.

Specific: The best goals are the ones that you will always be able to determine where you stand in relation to the goal. The goal should then have a clearly defined fail state as well as state that will let you know when you have crossed the finish line. Specific goals are also going to be much easier to chart out over time as their specificity will lend to clear sub-goals that can be linked to their success or failure.

Measurable: Appropriate goals are those which can be clearly defined between a set of points, one which indicates success and the other which indicates failure. Especially when you are first starting, it is important always to choose goals that will allow you to clearly know when you are drifting off track and when you are making progress.

Attainable: Good goals are always realistic to ensure that they are attainable and not simply an eternal carrot on a stick. There is a difference between easy goals and attainable ones. With easy goals, success is assured from the beginning and attaining them leads to few rewards. Attainable goals may take extensive planning and lots of hard work, but they are always more rewarding.

Relevant: It is important that the goal you choose is relevant to your current situation. Relevance is key to turning the SMART goal system from a one-time thing into a pattern and eventually a life-long habit that you can rely on to help you meet the challenges of life no matter what they may be.

Timely: SMART goals are those that have a clear deadline attached. Goals that don't have a clear timeframe for completion are goals that are less likely ever to be completed. Without a clear timetable, you can easily push off what you know you need to do indefinitely. Setting a timeframe will force you to confront what it is you want to do and work towards it. The timeframe you choose should be enough to make you hustle, but it doesn't need to be so tight that it is unrealistic.

Before you get ready to set your own goals, it is important to go ahead and do research so that you have a realistic idea of what it takes to accomplish the goal. This is important because if you set goals that you can't realistically expect to achieve in the timeframe that you have provided yourself, then you will be reinforcing negative habits that will make it even more difficult for you to try again in the future.

Conclusion

Congratulations on making it through to the end of *"Gastric Sleeve Bariatric Surgery Cookbook: The Complete Guide to Achieving Weight Loss Surgery Success with Over 100 Delicious Healthy Recipes."* I hope it was informative and able to provide you with all of the tools you need to achieve your weight loss goals. Just because you've finished this book doesn't mean there is nothing left to learn on the topic. Expanding your horizons is the only way to find the mastery you seek.

Now that you have made it through this book, you are likely feeling a little nervous (and hopefully excited) about the prospect of actually having the surgery. This is a perfectly natural response to what will certainly be a life-changing event. As there are so many steps ahead of you, it can be easy to get discouraged when thinking of just how far you are from the finish line. A great way to banish these thoughts is to stop thinking of what's ahead of you as a sprint and start thinking of it as a marathon. Slow and steady wins the race.

While every effort was made to ensure this book was as factual as possible, it is important to keep in mind that everyone is different which means your Doctor should have the final say on every step of your recovery. Likewise, it is important to always be on the side of caution to avoid accidentally doing more harm to yourself than good.

Finally, if you found this book helpful and insightful for your journey, please do leave a review on Amazon. This will help everyone else who is in a similar situation to you and feeling just as nervous about their journey.

Thank you.

Bibliography

- Bariatric Surgery Recipes. Retrieved from https://mayoclinichealthsystem.org/-/media/local-files/eau-claire/documents/medical-services/bariatric-surgery/bariatric-surgery-recipes.pdf?la=en&hash=D624574B942C016AF80E55554A2C8AE38234D8D2

- Wagner, S. (2017). Pureed and Soft Recipes Archives -. Retrieved from https://www.foodcoach.me/category/recipes/bariatricsoftrecipes/

- High Protein Dinner Recipes that are Bariatric Friendly | Bari Life. (2017). Retrieved from https://www.barilife.com/blog/high-protein-dinner-recipes-bariatric-friendly/

- Perfect Low-Sugar Smoothies - Bariatric Cookery. (2016). Retrieved from https://www.bariatriccookery.com/perfect-lowsugar-smoothies

- Soups Archives - Bariatric Foodie. Retrieved from https://www.bariatricfoodie.com/category/bariatric-recipes/soup/

- 12 Fruit Smoothies that solve your Bariatric Protein Dilemma. Retrieved from https://www.bariatriceating.com/2014/05/12-fruit-smoothies-that-solve-your-bariatric-protein-dilemma/

Made in the USA
San Bernardino, CA
30 December 2019